Dedication

Babaji - Belo

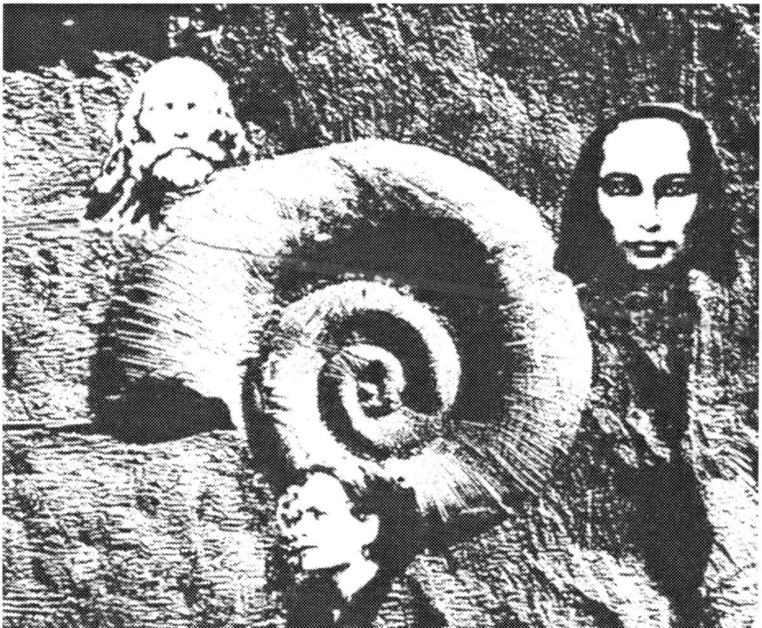

Acknowledgments

I was blessed by Babaji to write a book called 'The Path', a true gift from my Master and guru. He entrusted me with a task beyond my wildest dreams, which has been accomplished with the Blessing of God.

Thank you Dr Christian Kobau and Kornelia & Bernhard Wallner, devotees of Babaji, who, without their help and knowledge of reproducing the images to their optimum effect, 'The Path' would surely have taken ten times longer to materialise into print. Some of the images were taken from Christian's own book, 'The power of Your Healing Thoughts', which includes 2 DVD's containing a lecture; slideshow; healing sounds with gongs & crystal bowls, and poetry. Christian gave without thought of the work it created for himself and he moved at lightning speed. His was an example I aspire to. Special credit should be given to Mag Günter Jost who did the computer graphics for Christian. Please see Christian's web-site: www.kobau.at

Some of the images were also produced by Kornelia and Bernhard Wallner, whom I had the pleasure of meeting at Babaji's ashram. The front cover was taken from their work on The Six Days of Creation, which took 25 years to complete and is set to the music of Joseph Haydn. It is a spectacular piece of inspired work. Much work was put in by Kornelia on producing images for 'The Path' and I know that the loving energies produced by her work will be returned ten-fold. Kornelia and Bernhard can be contacted on e-mail: foto.wallner@aon.at

The Path

"I am the cry on the mountain. Come on my path.
Come unto me."

Maha Avatar Babaji

Emerald Giorgio

THE PATH

Library of Congress Catalogue No.2007046822

First Published in the UK by
Paul Mould Publishing
15 Standish Grove, Boston, Lincolnshire PE21 9EA
www.GetPublished.com
In association with
Empire Publishing Service
P.O. Box 1344, Studio City, CA 91614-0344
www.ppeps.com

A CIP Catalogue record for this book is available either from the British Library or, as below, from the US Library of Congress.

Simultaneously published in
Australia, Canada, Germany, UK, USA

Printed in Great Britain

First Printing 2007

Giorgio, Emerald.
The path / by Emerald Giorgio.
p.cm.
ISBN-13: 978-1-58690-067-0
1. Babaji--Teachings. 2. Yoga, Kriya. 3. Hindu parables. I. Title.
BL1175 . B18G56 2007
294.5'43--dc22
2007046822

US 13 ISBN 978-1-58690-067-0
UK 13 ISBN 978-1-904959-59-5

Contents

Introduction

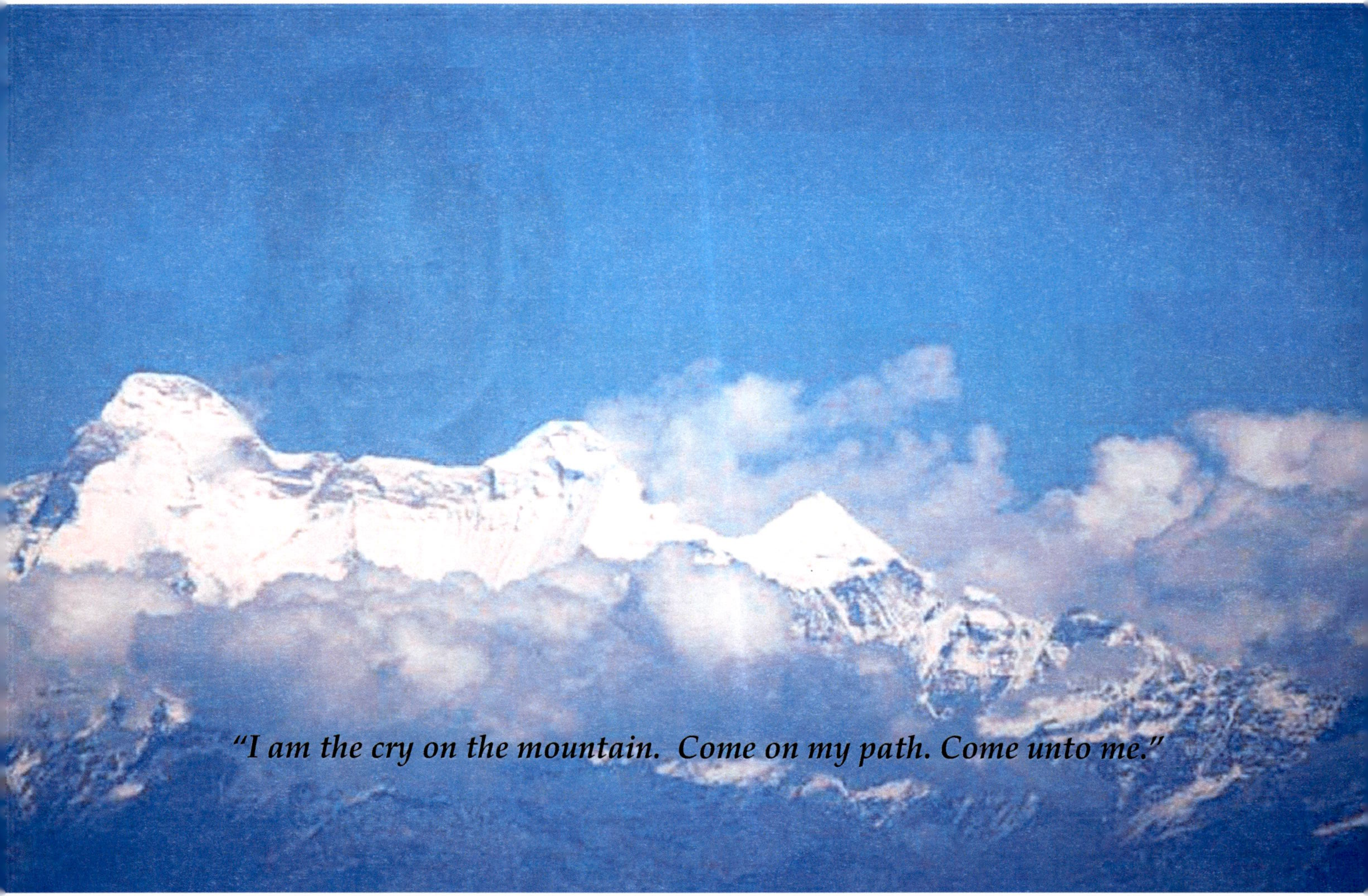
"I am the cry on the mountain. Come on my path. Come unto me."

Babaji's mission is to be the way which people can follow. He is the example on which we can model our lives. Throughout mankind's existence we have had such prophets and messengers of God sent to us in our hour of need to remind us when we go astray of what it is we are actually about. Well, let us start by listening to Babaji's words which are made simple by the luxurious repetition of God's name in all its forms of love.

The way is straight and winding, depending on how you approach yourself. Babaji is the highway but there are many possible detours we can take, all with the same end result but doubtless some more difficult than need be. The command to "Come unto me" can fill one with the absolute inability to move a single muscle in any direction, or speak any word in response, but he steadfastly repeats and repeats his words of encouragement, whilst oozing God's Love from every fibre of his being. Be comforted in the knowledge that he is here for us now. He is the listener's saviour. No sin will be left to fester within you if you follow his example, the way towards rejoicement.

Babaji is a herbalist and lover of nature with her boundless store of cures for all ails. He is also a doctor with a keen understanding of all things scientific, be it astrophysics, Einstein's Theory of Relativity or the psychology of man, but he goes beyond the face value of understanding and explains how everything is placed in the order of life and ultimately sourced from the Living God, our Creator. No matter what your question is, he will have an answer ready for you in some form at the appropriate level of spiritual growth and healing, depending on what your individual need is.

Babaji's name is intrinsically associated with the science of Kriya Yoga and he has passed his knowledge on to countless people from all walks of life, both from the East and from the West. Some of these people are well known spiritual leaders themselves, such as Paramahansa Yogananda, the author of 'Autobiography of a Yogi', who received the instruction from Babaji to leave India and go to the West to propagate the way towards our Living God, including the kriyas. Babaji told him to build a bridge between the East and West, to aid relations between our countries. This, Paramahansa Yogananda did. Another spiritual leader and guru to receive the kriya initiations from Babaji was Sai Baba, who resides in the south of India with a large international following of devotees. Omraan Michael Ivanhov, too, received the kriya initiations, spending some time with Babaji before leaving for California and founding the 'White Brotherhood' in the West.

The knowledge of the kriya yoga system of utilising the life's force within the body was revealed by Babaji some 800 years ago to Shankarachariya, to whom he was a guide at that time. The kriyas enable an individual to grow towards God, living a clean life according to the laws of nature, in the manner given to us by our Lord God in the Ten Commandments. Our rewards for living this path through God, as against our man-made laws, is the bliss of rejoicement in our hearts and the release of all things burdensome in our struggle to survive.

The Origin of Man

Even if you have started to look at your past life experiences, your ancestors and old belief systems, there still remains the question, "But where do I come from? Where did I exist before all this?" You just know you are whom you are.

Babaji sat on the steps of his ashram, draped in his plain white chola. The sun shone down on him as his smile also shone down on his devotees. They were waiting for his next words, sometimes aimed at a single person, but mostly for all. He sometimes looked at one person yet aimed his words at another. He was so clever at ensuring each person got his message from God. Oh, how his love pervaded those who listened and those who merely wished to be close to him. His words may seem to come ad hoc, but there was always a reason and system to his discourses which came in a circle of information, depending on the needs of the devotees present at the time. His devotees came and went. Some stayed for a few hours, days or months, and almost certainly returned if they had the ears for his words.

As he sat in the sun, taking in all its energies, a kriya of the sun, he began to tell his devotees about their creation, how the Word banged and all universes and galaxies came into being.

"In the beginning was the Word, says the Holy Bible, and this is so. We are given a life to experience all things, a 3-day life, a life in which we take 3 births," said Babaji, and this was the point where the devotees were to begin to take note of the differences in the teachings of our ancestors and those of the Maha Avatar Babaji. It was best to put aside all man-made beliefs and allow Babaji's wisdom to pervade your heart, soul and mind with his message of the One Living God, Whom we should worship. No matter what your ethnic background, religious or non-religious faith, his words fell easily into place in your own jigsaw puzzle of life.

"You are nothing but cosmic dust, come from the Heavenly Father down on to this Mother Earth," Babaji said. "Our first, original birth was in heaven. We were created in the mass of all things by the Word of God. There was a time when all spirits gathered together before their Creator and made a promise to always worship Him, and only Him. There were to be no other gods or idols whom we should bow down before, and in order that we should remember this oath, God gave us His messengers who would remind us. These messengers are the prophets who come down to earth to show us the path again and again, especially when we are at the most blind part of our progress, when mankind's detours off the path are corrupt and veering towards a dead end, because we have made gods of ourselves.

"As we look at the sun we see its glow and believe it to be much bigger than our beautiful Mother Earth. Our scientists tell us that it is billions times bigger than earth." Babaji paused before giving the next revelation.

"The sun is nothing. It is only the smallest of cosmic atoms which was diffused by the Finger of God, ignited to give life to mankind." Again, he paused so that his devotees had the opportunity to absorb the magnitude of this revelation. "God made everything in duality: first individuality, then duality, to be returned to individuality. This will be our third birth, our resurrection." Babaji then continued to relate the truth of mankind's second birth, how he came into being on Mother Earth.

"Our Heavenly Father or the Invisible Planet, is the aurum or sky surrounding Mother Earth. He sends his milk down on the Milky Way and thus we are created from this cosmic dust, when our physical mother and father are blessed by nature with a child, boy or girl. When we die, we return once more to the 'deep freezer' of the Heavenly Father to await reincarnation. Our spirit resides in the womb of Mother Earth before we continue with our life's experiences in another life span.

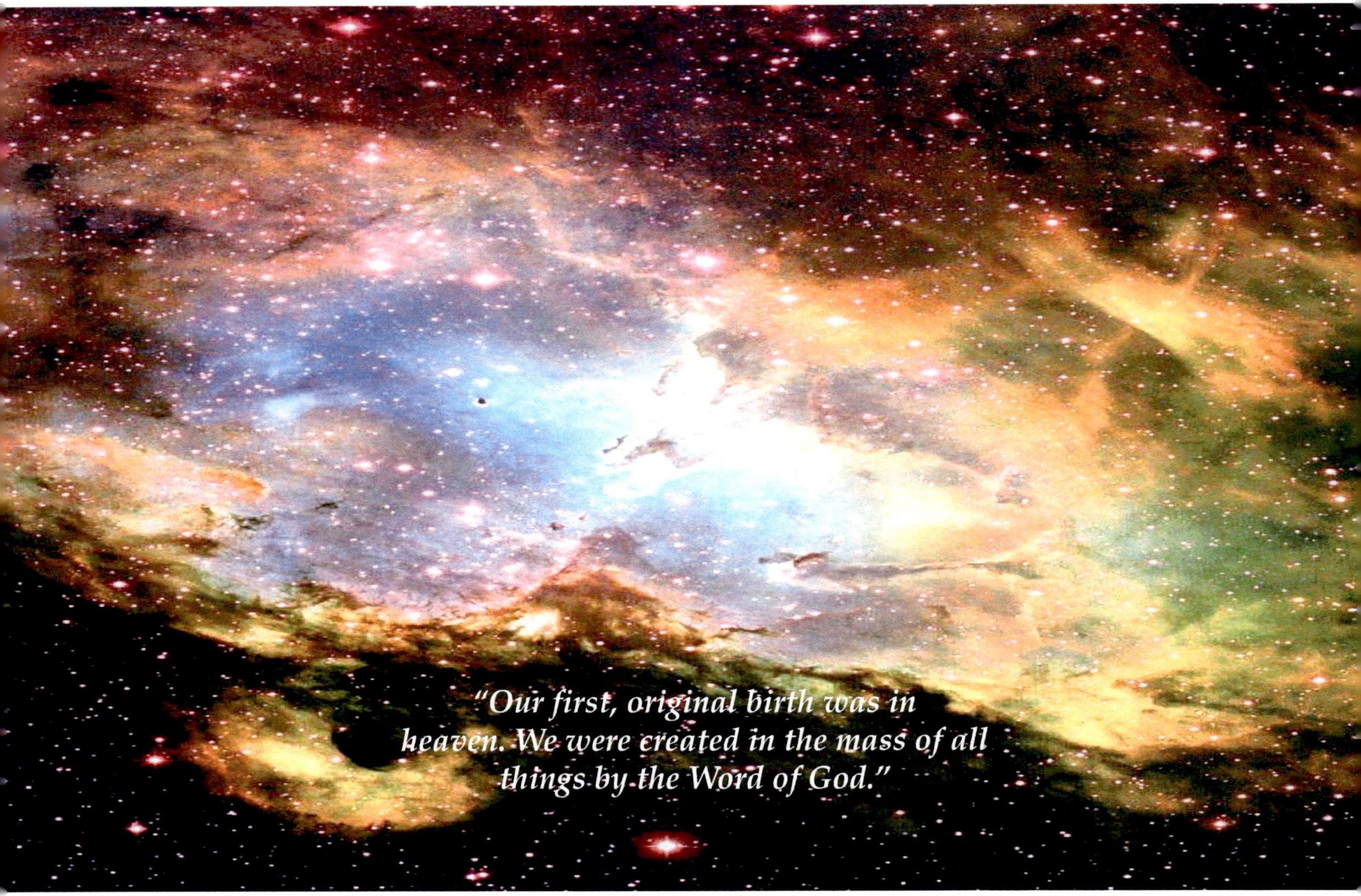
"Our first, original birth was in heaven. We were created in the mass of all things by the Word of God."

"Our physical body is nothing but the culmination of our ancestors' karmic debts, as well as those of our own making. Our body merely consists of our karmic mass and our soul is separate from this dreamy way of life we call existence. Our soul and spirit are geared to remember God, to worship only the One Omniscient Living God, as we walk the path of our earthly existence."

Babaji considered the needs of his devotees before him and once more flowed into action with his words. His animated face and free-flowing prayer to the Lord God continued at all times as he spoke and paused. The sea of faces gazed up in wonderment at both Babaji and his revelations.

"Now, I am going to teach you the Tattva Gyana, the knowledge of existence. We are created in symmetry with the Lord God and our bodies contain all galaxies, continents, mountains, rivers and oceans. There is symmetry and duality in the way we are created. We have two eyes, two ears, two nostrils, two hands and two feet. This is the Divine Father and Divine Mother in us and the Blessing of the Lord God. We have within us a lake of holy water, which is in the pineal gland at the top of our head, also known as the sahasradhara chakra. From this lake flow two rivers, the Ganges and the Yamuna. They flow down the front of your body and coincide at the points known as the chakras. These islands are the points where all desires and wishes come from and the rivers create the solutions to progress the sentiments of our own making.

"Mother Earth's centrifugal point is within us, known as the kalachakram. The kalachakram spins in the opposite direction to that of Mother Earth. Our spine is the same axis as Mother Earth's, and the tenure of our kalachakram is the time machine, also known as the Book of Life, where a full account of our deeds and actions is recorded.

"The Divine Nectar is flowing down within us, cleaning all points of pilgrimage where we visit during meditation in order to cleanse the heats and desires. When meditating, take the chi, or life's force, above the lower realms of earthly living and work the time machine in the opposite direction. This is the way back to God and God-realisation. If the rivers of life are left to flood and flow without attention, then all is lost in this life span. The flow eventually cools, icing up, and the life spark is taken back into the realms of the Heavenly Father for reprocessing, once the Book of Life is accounted for in this life time. This is the process of reincarnation, the playing out of karma.

"So, when the water pours down, it stimulates our sun and moon. Our Mother Earth and moon within do not only revolve around our sun, but the sun is also orbiting with Mother Earth in this solar galaxy, and this solar galaxy is travelling in a big circle around another galaxy. The holy water generates our seed which sprout like trillions and trillions of springs flowing down to the tips of our toes. This is the knowledge of the Tattva Gyana." Babaji waited before continuing with the concept of the One Living God.

"Who believes in Darwin's Theory of Evolution, that man evolved from the ape-man? Who believes that we are nothing but the chance product of two beings getting together? Has there not to be more to this earthly existence than eating, sleeping and the passing pleasures of worldly desires?" His devotees waited for his answers to these fundamental questions.

"There is only the One Omniscient Living Power of God, the Ultimate and Infinite, the Alpha and the Omega, the Loving Creator of all things. He sparked the sun with the tip of His Finger and all things were created in that moment when the Word banged, when God spoke. When all spirits got together and made their promise to God to always worship Him and only Him, He gave us the gift of our 'made-easies', the prophets and messengers, to help us on our path.

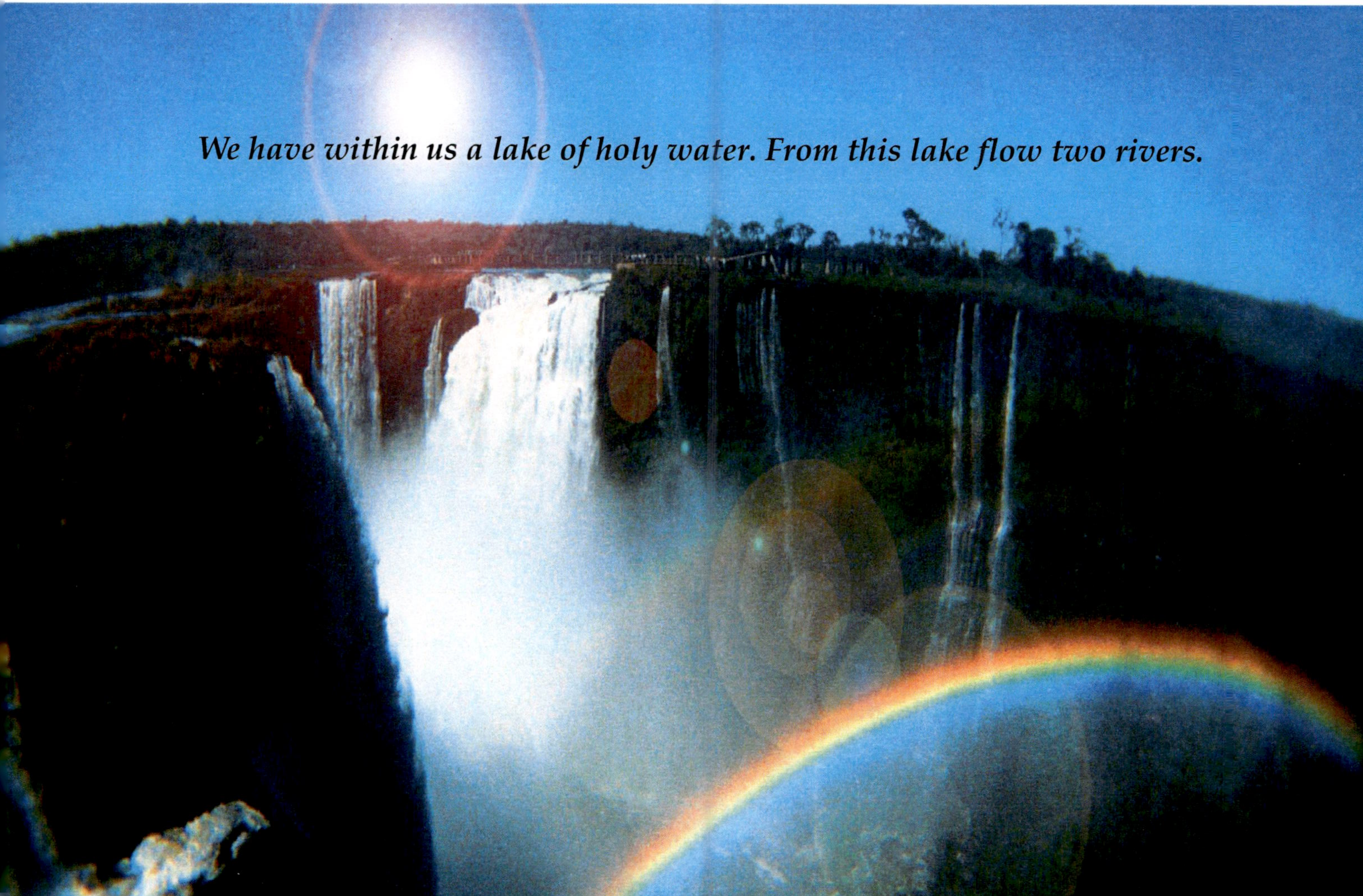

We have within us a lake of holy water. From this lake flow two rivers.

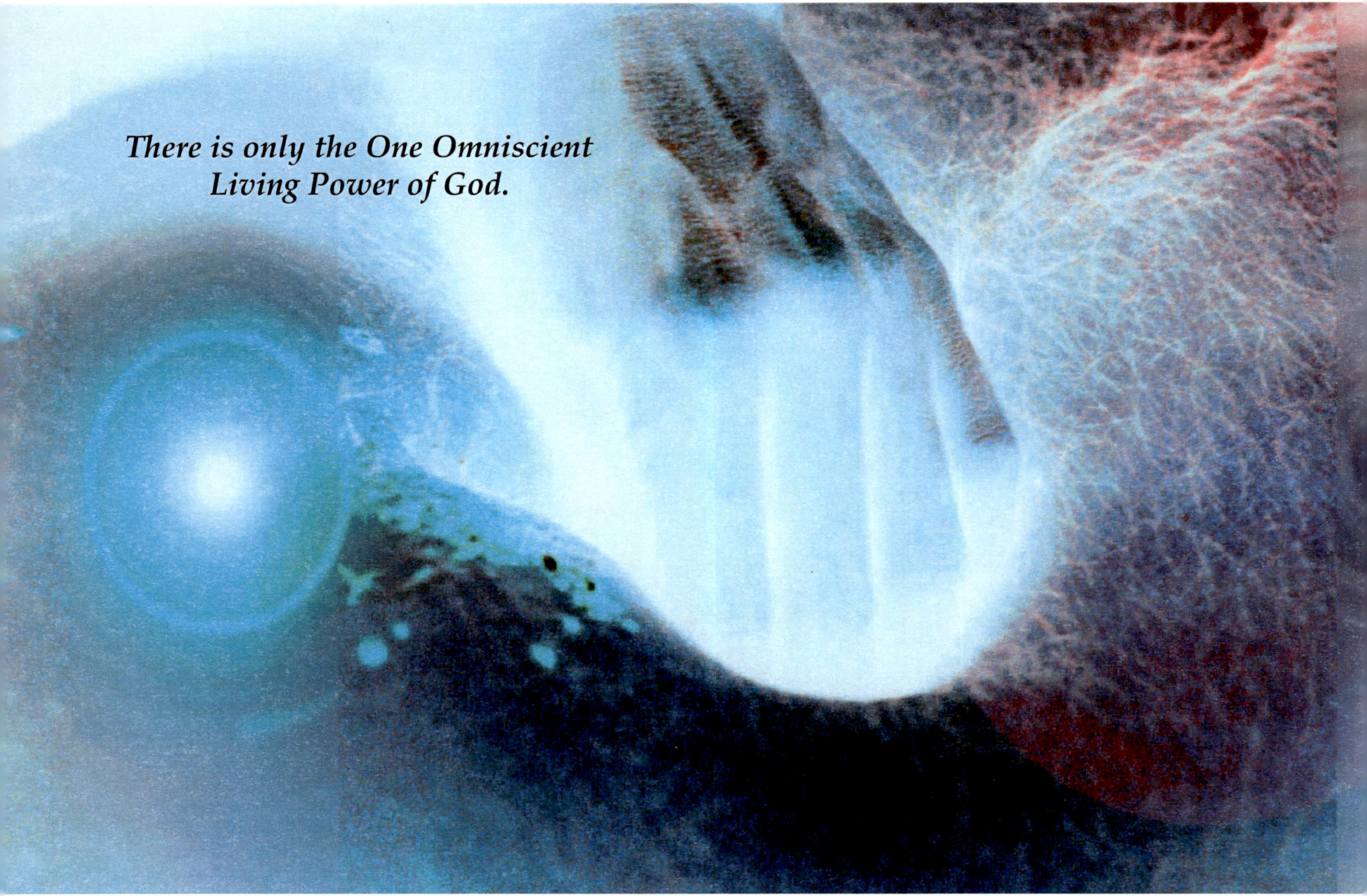
*There is only the One Omniscient
Living Power of God.*

"In God there is all things, all qualities of existence, and we are made in direct symmetry with Him. The difference between mankind and the rest of the Lord God's Creation is this: He gave to mankind the animals, plants and trees to beautify and balance life on dear Mother Earth. The difference is the wisdom inside us, which we are to search for and utilise when walking the path of life. All of God's Creation has its own intellect by which it conducts itself. Each wild animal has its own intellect or instinct by which it is able to exist. Each plant, tree, flora and fauna has its own intellect by which it can procreate and continue its existence on this earth. But the Lord God blessed man with the potential wisdom to know what is right and what is wrong, so that we are able to make our way on the Path of Righteousness. He also took away from mankind the instinct of survival of the fittest, and this is the difference between us and our fellow creatures on Mother Earth.

"Our origin is not from the ape-man. We are God's Creation, made by the blessing of the Divine Father and the Divine Mother."

Babaji completed his teaching for the day. The information was enough for his devotees to digest this day.

What is Inside Your Sun?

Babaji stepped out into the full sun, took a deep breath as he raised his hands up unto the sky and smiled, saying in a loud voice, "Dear God, thank You for the sunshine this day. We thank You for each and every gift Thy hast given this day. Oh, how Great Thou Art. Thou art the Greatest and Most Bounteous. Let us remember always to bow down towards You in honour of Thy Greatness."

The day had a good feel to it and the crowd were in good humour. There was a general hub-hub in the air and there was an expectation hanging heavily amongst Babaji's devotees. It was a mixed crowd, each small clutch of people with their own issues and needs, but Babaji was never phased. He always took his time and allowed the flow of God's energies to take its full toll, before venturing towards the people. He weighed up the situation and then started the engine. He was the engine driver and he started the forward motion of the locomotive.

"Let there be rejoicement this day. Lift up your hearts and pay tribute to the Lord God Whom has blessed us with this day. He has opened the portals of the sun energy upon us and we are blessed," Babaji commenced.

The sun shone down and down, lighting up all things at varying degrees, depending upon whose shadow was cast where. The light reflected and deflected, and the people's faces glowed as the residue of the sun's rays touched them. There was a definite magic in the air as Babaji cranked up the engine and gathered momentum. The people were going on a magical mystery tour and were to follow the brightly coloured umbrella that Babaji led with.

"I want you to close your eyes, look up into your third eye and look INSIDE. Let us see what is inside your sun." The crowd fell quiet and stilled themselves. They felt the rhythm of the locomotive humming and vibrating at different resonances. They were now totally still and sat in calmness as the machine of their collective vibrations

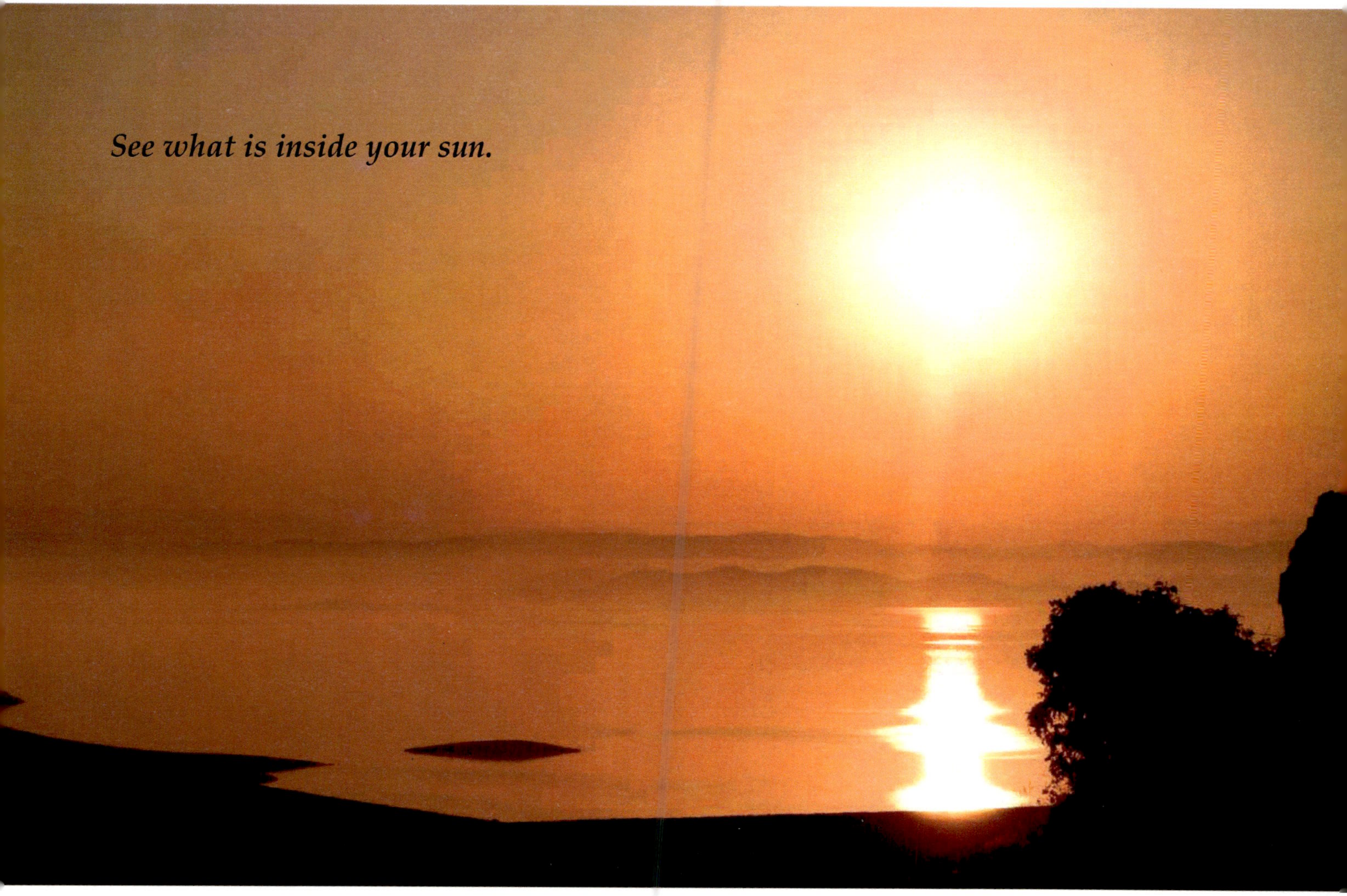
See what is inside your sun.

was worked by the Master. Their breathing was relaxed and each person bore a gentle smile upon his face.

Their sun loomed closer and closer, and soon all they could sense was a beautiful aura within, where some dared to venture. They found only peace and a feeling of being sustained. They were about to experience their truth within. Their sun was about to reveal the truth behind his solar energy. The engine purred and in the background was another humming vibration, which intertwined with that of the locomotive. Oh, how impossible it seemed that each rhythm could work together, weaving a cloth of many colours. The tattoo seemed so complex but it wove with such ease.

Those people who were able to reach such heights gathered yet more momentum, and their inner motors moved onwards and upwards. Babaji observed their well-oiled pistons flying. The sun gave way to the void behind and there was the jewell in the sky, the Invisible Planet, the Golden Planet, from whence we came. Babaji's words came back to the people as they beheld the Divine Father's totality.

"You are nothing but cosmic dust, come down from the Heavenly Father on the vehicle of the Milky Way to this Mother Earth. You come from the Heavenly Father's deep freezer of spirits who await their time on earth, returning and returning, each time with more pages of their Book of Life written up. As you drop down once more with your balance sheet set to rebalance with the Blessing of God, observe the simplicity of good living, or God-living, before the veils wrap around you and you find yourself in the arms of your earthly mother."

The people who were able to see, noted the two rivers flowing down from their heads, down into the oceans within their stomachs. They saw their water's life flow into the oceans within and heard a sound. They did not know what the sound was, but they knew it was a vital part of their existence.

"I can hear something," said one small voice in wonderment. "What can it be that sounds so sweet?"

"Oh, child of mind," responded Babaji, "what you hear is the Song of God within you. Let it ring through every sinew of your being. Let it flow out into the universe. Let God be the receiver of your prayers. He is the best listener. Declare your colours of life and worship the One Omniscient Living God."

So, the people shone their lights towards their One God and the sun shone upon them. The sun had revealed its truth, its place in the whole of things.

The Light of Mohammed is the Logos

"The Light of Mohammed is the Logos and he showed the sunna, his living example, as the path to God."

The sun was rising as a new day was presenting itself. What blessings would the Almighty Living God bestow through Babaji on his children this day? Babaji had been in meditation for the last few hours and already he knew what it was that was needed. However, first he wished to hear the first call of the birds and see the first beam of sunlight, so that he could doubly feel the light in his heart. He felt the rejoicement of the first moments of the day and was sustained. He always liked these precious moments of quietude when he would realise the gifts from heaven above for himself, and he always remembered to give thanks and praise to his Lord God for everything, from the smallest chirping of the birds to the laughing faces of the local children.

"Oh, Lord God, thank You so much for all that Thou hast given me this day forward. You are the most Merciful and Compassionate. I bow down in service to Thee. Let me be a fine instrument of Thy Truth. Give me the wherewithal, dear Lord." Then he heard the soft whispering in his ear.

"Dear son, the people today need to be reminded of the Dharma, the real path to Me; how to live the perfection of man's daily life, clean of heart and clean of body."

Babaji moved forward to the jasmine bush, breathed in its heavenly scent, and knew that all angels were with him this day, a minimum of one angel per person would attend his ashram.

It was not long before the people started to arrive, in small groups as well as those who had travelled alone to be within his aura. As they approached him, each man, woman and child paid respect to their mentor and Guru, which he accepted with such grace and ease. The perfume of the jasmine wafted through the crowd which was now filling to goodly numbers. Time was often forgotten by Babaji as he flowed with the Almighty's timelessness within him. The people were patient and enjoyed the ambience of the developing day. The angels gathered muster as they were invited one by one by Babaji to work with the Lord God's wishes that his children would hear their individual call. The cool, golden light of the angels permeated the masses and there was laughter in the air.

"The Divine Father and Divine Mother have blessed you with this life," Babaji began. "Please do not waste this wonderful opportunity to progress down your path of God's opening to you. You have the will inside, and can make use of every breath you take to inspire and call others to His Way. Let there be light amongst all men. Let there be love towards all living matter. Love thy Mother Earth as she gives so abundantly to her inhabitants. Live thy lives according to nature and the Laws of God. You have been given these laws through the prophet, Moses, who dedicated his life to helping mankind see the light and knowledge within each and every soul. Look inside for the right direction to turn, every footstep you take, every breath you inhale. Surely there can be no mistaking the Song of God when it croons the words and melody of the Almighty and Eternal God.

"Follow not the laws of man-made instigation. These laws are only for the furtherance of his own man-made idols and gods. The lords and gods of man work merely for his own power, money and worldly desires. He lures you in with the pleasures of the flesh, when all the time you need to be above these wishes of the lower instincts.

"If you believe in the Eternal God, then you get eternity. If you believe in this matter, then you live in this mass. If you live above this mass, then you will rise above this mass."

Babaji looked down with love in his eyes at his devotees as they integrated this revelation into their hearts and minds. He knew he had made his mark this day, but would still go on and on until his words could be no more. He paused a short while for his devotees to settle once more…

The Way of The Lord

Babaji saw the mood of his making grow into something different. The people were responding to his words of advice.

"But, how is it possible not to obey the law of the land, Babaji?" said one old man, who had the experience of hard living etched around his eyes and mouth. The lines of a life of poverty and hard labour had made their mark, but he never faltered in his devotion to his Master and Guru, Babaji. "We must surely pay our taxes and live within a civil society, which means spending time and our hard-earned money on things we might not otherwise wish." The crowd rippled in agreement with the wisdom of what their elder had voiced, an echo of their own feelings of doubt.

"You are quite right, my son," said Babaji, but there is a better way of seeing to the needs of others and still living the clean life. In the first placed we should always love our neighbour as we do ourselves. This means contributing to a community which sustains thyself.

"The Laws of God came to Moses through the Baptism of Fire on Mount Thor. Moses came down the mountain side equipped with all answers to this very fundamental need of mankind. Man needs to know which way to conduct himself within society but, most importantly, he needs to find the balance between right living and 'conforming'. In this case, the word 'conforming' is used with an absolute looseness of man-made thinking. Weave the cloth with God's Word written in every thread and thou shalt not falter. If you love and worship only the One Living God and not the stuff of thine ancestors, who have passed on to you the misinterpretations of their wrong thinking, you will not falter.

"Love only the Almighty, Loving, Living and One Omniscient, Eternal God. Praise His Name as you walk to the market place or as you carry the results of your toil to sell to your fellow man. Imbue the Name of God in all your travails, and only good can come out of thy actions. This is the truth, the Law of God. If you think that something is not right in the community, pray to the Almighty God:

Dear Lord and Creator of mankind,
forgive our foolish ways.
Reclothe us in our rightful minds
in purer lives Thy service find,
and in deeper reverence praise.

Let us trust Thy gracious calling,
and drop our strains and stress,
as we rise up to follow Thee, oh Lord.
We ask that You liberate our souls,
that we may feel the beauty of Thy Peace.
Calm the heats of our desire
with the coolness of Thy Balm."

(Words taken loosely from a hymn by Quaker poet, John Greenleaf Whittier)

"Babaji, that is most soothing," said another devotee from the crowd. This time it was the voice of a grandmother with her family sitting beside her, "but, we need to teach our children the way of things as they are lured towards the trappings of the material world outside. How do we stop them from turning down the wrong direction, when all they desire is the apparent abundance of man's market place?" Babaji's response was swift.

"If you keep your home in accordance with God's bounteous laws, the love of the Lord God will penetrate every corner of your abode and touch the hearts and minds of the youngsters who are vulnerable to the attractions of false gods, the gods of man's own making. Remember that it is God's Law which offers abundance, not the false promises of man. Man thinks himself to be a self-god and does not see the lush bounty of the Almighty. Man has blinded himself to the point of no return, and I am here to help you redirect yourself on the Path of the Lord God. God's Law is unfailing. He takes nothing from man. He only gives, gives and gives.

"Be open to the gifts of nature, the Divine Mother. She is the Love of God in material form. The abundance of her wealth is here for mankind to enjoy without the need to stress. If you give life to your fellow-man, then life will be given to you. If you offer succour to the starving man at your door, you will be given succour. If you smile at the down-turned eyes of a passing stranger, then you will be smiled upon by a fleeting sunbeam or the twinkling of a bright star in the night sky. God's Law is Finite in its Infinite nature. It is just, and you shall receive all that is due to you according to how you behave in this life. Your own unconditional love within the family unit will pervade the day to day living of both the young and the aged. Remember to praise the Heavenly Father in gratitude for his fortitude and succour."

Without realising it, the people were gifted with a piece of fortitude to take with them in their daily lives. They were enlightened in the Way of the Lord and were empowered by the words of their Babaji. They bestowed him with gifts of sweets made by their own hand, and all was distributed in the manner of their Guru and friend. Oh, how he was loved by his following of devotees from afar and wide. His loving vibrations reached out into the universe, calling the cry on the mountain.

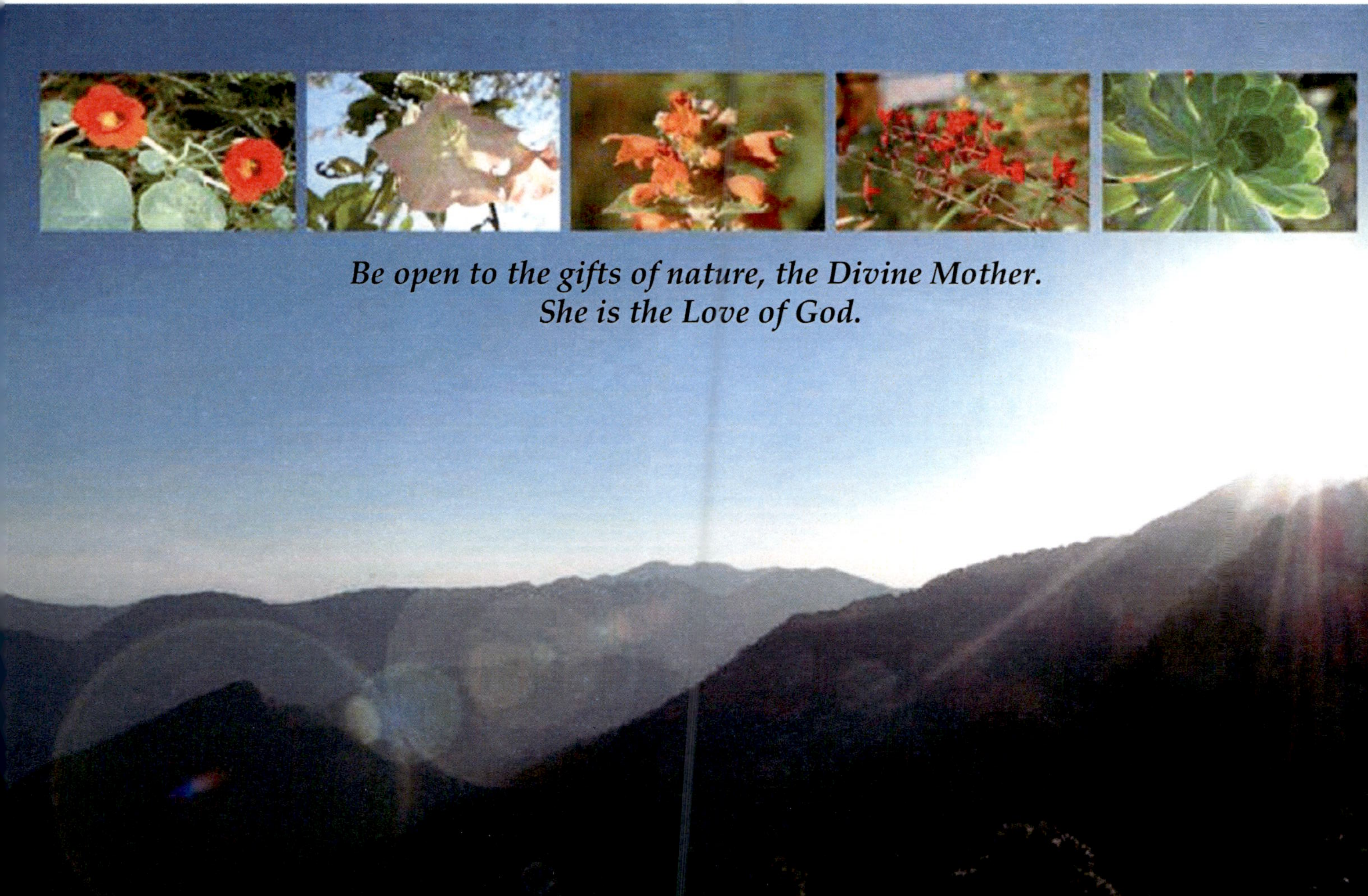

Be open to the gifts of nature, the Divine Mother.
She is the Love of God.

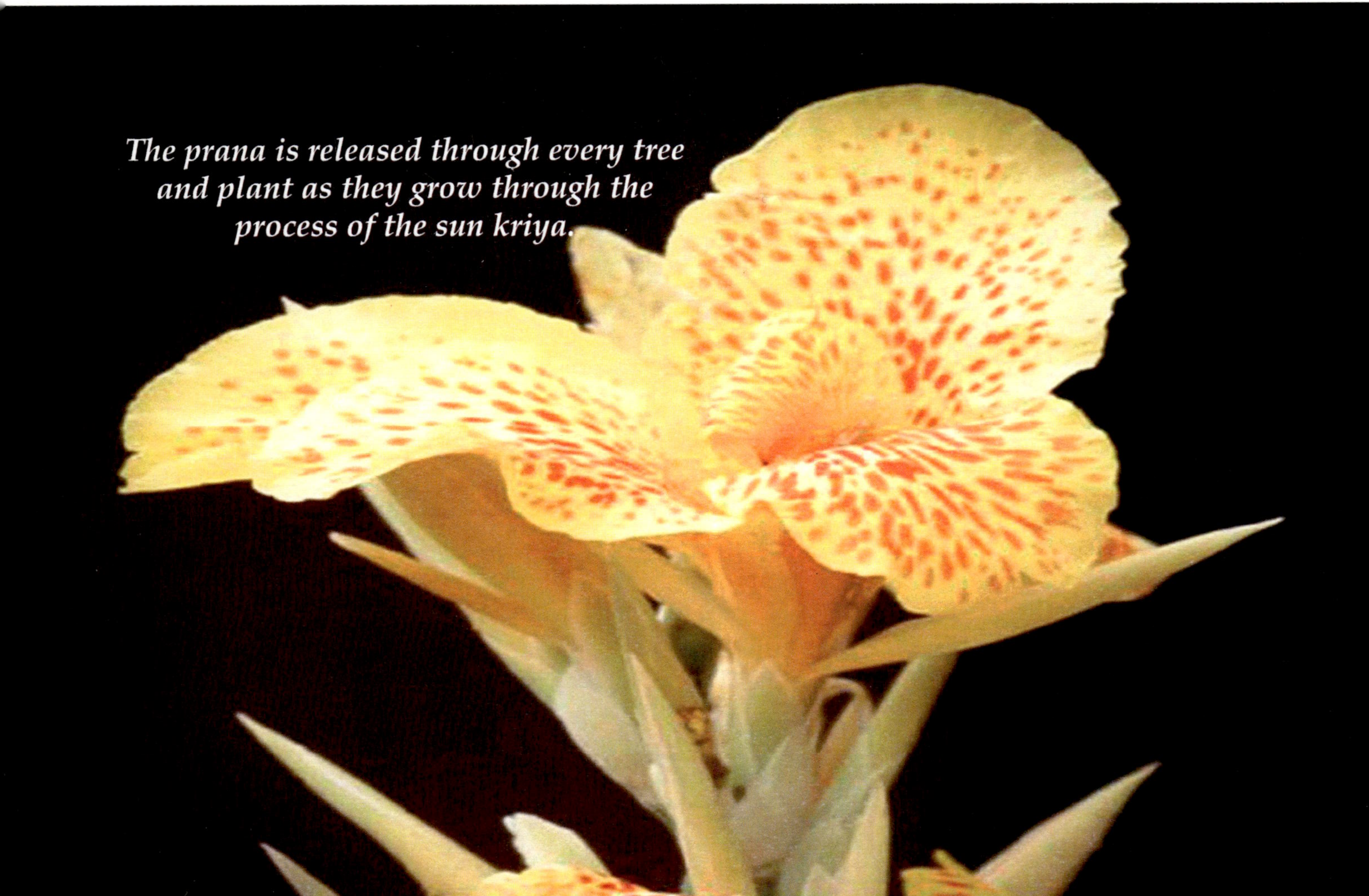
The prana is released through every tree and plant as they grow through the process of the sun kriya.

The Essence of Life

The call of the day had begun and Babaji was ready. He was following his own heart and mind into the wilderness of the density of the outside material world. He was arming himself with God's life-force, the essence of life. He took his first deep breath, drawing it up and up and up until he had the fire burning in all parts of his body. The air (prana) was his food, the Food of God, and he was sustained. Babaji was the bringer into this world of the kriya breathing system and had ensured that its powers were kept pure by passing on the knowledge to those who were of right mind, body and spirit. He loved to see the spiritual growth of those who steadfastly practiced the techniques of the kriyas, be it in small, bite-size pieces, or, for those of more robust constitution, the more enduring regime of practice. He watched carefully over his disciples as they huffed and puffed their first attempts, and saw them progress to a serene state of consciousness. He would adjust their techniques here and there until they were able to follow their own inner wisdom with the kriyas. He was the Master of the kriya yoga and would leave it to God's Will as to where the knowledge was dispersed throughout the world. He trusted in His Way of Things. No man-made law was required to 'protect' the kriyas.

Babaji walked down the ashram steps towards the City of Nainital, towards the local market place. His people would soon hear that his presence was in their vicinity rather than in the peaceful grounds of his trees and flowers. He was fleet of foot and with each step he left a prayer for the next person to receive as they followed in his loving vibration. The night had known rainfall and the air was fresh with the smell of Mother Earth rising up into Babaji's nostrils. He breathed in deep the energy of her blessings and noted the dews of water resting on the tiny flowers clinging to the steep slopes of the path down to the lake. The rainbow refractions of the drops as they sat on the delicate petals gave off all God's colour into the environment of man. Babaji was filled with gratitude and gave thanks to the Almighty God for the gifts of the moment.

"Oh, Lord God, Thou art the Greatest, Who never fails to light up the day. I give thanks to You, dear Lord, for your continuous flow of abundance, as I fill myself with the prana of life. Your treasure trove is rich, indeed."

Babaji, too, was beginning to be acknowledged by the local town's people, who bent down to touch his feet in love and honour of his presence. Some continued on their way as they had work to do, but others followed, knowing there would be words to hear if they were lucky that day. He stopped by the willow tree, grown big with age and experience. The water's edge of Lake Naini lapped as the song of nature rang out in total harmony with the day. The birds bellowed out their song, too. Who would believe that such sound could emit from such a small being? It was a miracle, indeed. A seat was found for Babaji by a tradesman whose shop was nearby, and he made himself comfortable for the next hours.

Men, women and children now surrounded their beloved Babaji, some with mere curiosity, but the majority in eager anticipation. Babaji commenced gently into his discourse. He knew it was important for his people to understand the ease with which their lives could be lived. He wanted to show them that things need not be so difficult, if only they would turn away from the worshipping of man's dead gods and idols. Never had he been so intent in his mission to show his devotees the burden of their worldly ways and how easy it was to follow him on the Path of the One, Eternal, Omniscient God.

There was a reason for Babaji choosing the location of the willow tree. The fact that there was space around it was only of added benefit. Its roots spread along the surface of the ground as its branches swept downwards over his loving countenance. The tree was a part of Babaji's aura now, blending in its own healing essence with that of his. Willow was for the resentment and gall. Its flexing ability to retain strength in any compromising situation was exactly what Babaji required. He was sure of his friend, who sheltered him from the unbidden energies of negativity. The scene was set and his words rolled out from his heart and soul.

"The prana of life is the Food of God," he began. "It is to be brought into all aspects of life, be it for the sake of an easy day's work or, more importantly, for the worship of the Lord God in all His forms. The prana is released through every tree and plant as they grow through the process of the sun kriya. They are God's living example of how the energies can be utilised to the fullest as they bow their heads in reverence towards their Living Lord God. They are God's living example of how to enjoy His Essence of Life.

"God gave us everything. We are sustained and nothing is required for us to proceed in life. We have the clear knowledge of His assured existence. Our guidance is complete. We just have to obey God's Law and we shall succeed. Live for the Living God, the One, Almighty, Living God, Who hast no requirement of you except that you remember your way back to Him. He is the goal and once we get our footsteps on His Way, there will be no falling down. Dedicate every breath and footstep to the Elohim. Let the rhythm of His Name blend in the daily passing of time here on your Mother Earth. She is the Divine Mother who takes care of our every need. Speak to her when you are weary or weak of heart. She will give strength and empowerment to those in need. She is the Divine Mother and it is her job to care. It is this essence that needs to be encompassed in our own beings so that we, in return, also take care of our Mother Earth and her precious ecology of life. Live according to nature, the Law of God, and you will surely succeed in all things, from the tiniest of blessings received, to the magnitude of world-wide blessings. Make sure you spend time in the receiving mode. Note and give thanks to the Lord God for the blessings of each day and night. He is the Greatest and He is the Almighty, Eternal, Living God. Remember Him."

The Life of Cleanliness

Babaji stilled himself before taking a new tack with his words.

"If you live a clean life, the Law of God will naturally follow. You will attract all that is good towards you, affecting all creatures and beings of God's Creation around you. You will be a light for the Lord God and an instrument of His Will. Do good, think good, walk good and talk good, for the sake of the Universal Brotherhood. The Blessings of God are in profusion upon those whose mind is clear of mindless chatter and outer influences. Keep your own counsel and feel the rhythm of life, the Song of God, within your heart and soul. You are the chosen beings whom God watches from all quarters. Never think that you are alone. God is always with you and sees your every notion and motion. Keep still in the presence of the Glory of the Almighty God and you will hear His soft words whispering in your inner ear. It is His wish that you follow His Path, and as you tread the course, bring along with you those who need the earthly words of assurance that His Way is True. His Way is Eternal and He will provide the necessary cleansing energy for you."

Still, the people sat next to their Guru, Babaji. He had been in full flow and they were in receptive mood. The willow was working its magic and Babaji ebbed and flowed in direct resonance with the healing properties of Mother Nature. The gentle breeze caught hold of the willow's curtain of leaves and wafted her filigree of woven cloth over the whole mass of the crowd. They were enmeshed in the binding of the Divine Mother and felt only the love of their mentor, sifting into their finely tuned systems. Babaji had done his tweaking and adjusting of his people's receivers and amplifiers, and they could leave as and when they needed. Always they paid tribute to him before taking their leave, filled with the Food of God to help them on their way. The Will of the Almighty God was done. Babaji got up from his seat beneath the willow, and gave thanks and praise to the Lord for the lush provision of the day.

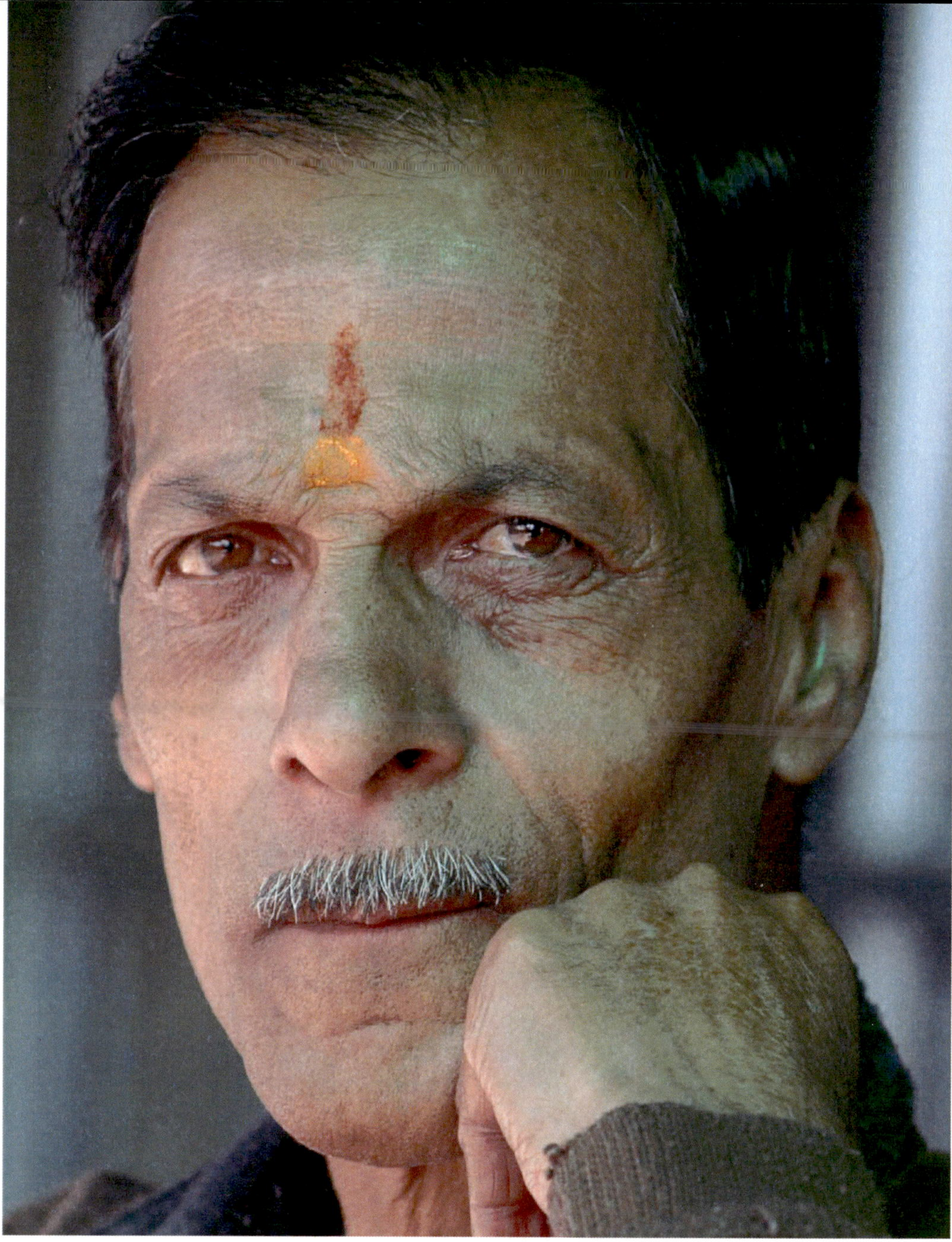

Do good, think good,
walk good and talk good.

The discourse had been received well and the angels dispatched the sentiments through their own unique waves of communication. They would reach the smallest of pin-holes in the hearts and minds of each man, woman and child, whose doubts might seek to 'protect' them from the dangers of unknown ground. God's Will Be Done.

One young man remained seated by Babaji's feet. He did not want to depart before asking what seemed to him to be a difficult question of his Guru. Babaji did not give any sign that he needed to return to his ashram with urgency although it was, indeed, the case.

"Yes, my son. What is it that you want?" he asked.

"Babaji, please tell me how to cleanse the karmas of my ancestors as well as those of my own doing. It seems such an impossible task for each person to do in this world. As soon as we have gained the forgiveness of our Lord God for our sins of the day, there are new sins committed in a split second of time."

Babaji did not pause. He just said, "Purify yourself by regular fasting. Only eat the living food, the food which has the essence of life, not the food which is corrupt with man's interference with nature. Man has no thought of the consequences of his progressive ways of eating. He feeds fowl and beast with the dead bones of his fellow man, the dead substances of man's making, leaving the food with no life's essence. This process will eventually filter through to your own body and you, yourself, will become a dead being. Rid yourself of man's thoughtless ways and cleanse yourself. Live according to the law of nature, eating clean, pure food. Be a good vegetarian and take in the goodness of plants and crops which have had the benefit of the sun energy. Receive the sun energy into your being by eating, breathing and thinking its energies.

"It is by the miracle of God's own creation that you are able to cleanse yourself of all karmas. I am your witness and shall be there at your Day of Reckoning. Do not fear that you are alone, my son. I am with you always and shall be with you when you account for your sins and those of your ancestors, written in your Book of Life."

The young man was appeased and thanked his Master, Babaji, for his words of wisdom. He knew he had received the blessing of Babaji as he made his way home that late afternoon.

Who Am I?
So I Am

Babaji was listening to the rhythm of Mother Earth's breath. She was only the Divine Mother of this small galaxy but her existence was paramount to mankind. Her song was ringing vibrantly in Babaji's heart and he could feel her earthy resonance filling his lungs, thymus and third eye. He saw her song emit in wave upon wave of higher and lower frequencies as they danced in and out of their rising and ebbing notes. He felt his own soul note begin to move towards that of the Divine Mother. It was the colour of God and he knew it to be true. It also gave off semi-rhythms and quarter-rhythms to blend in with the sacred geometry of his Mother Earth. They were at one: In and out, in and out. Babaji felt the bliss of his Heavenly Mother.

Another day was dawning and he began to stir from his deep meditation. Slowly, he brought himself back into the four walls of his chamber until he felt the ground beneath him. He would have to move quickly if he was to catch the first rays of the sun glistening on the mountain tops. He was not to be disappointed that day. It was a new September matinee of the dawn chorus and the mists accompanied the bright beams of light, shafting across the Nainital Valley.

Today he would show the Swan Kriya breath to the new arrivals from the West. They showed good potential and he was eager to progress them before they returned to their homeland. Western people were being attracted to the East more and more and always took back a wealth of knowledge to their friends back home. The word was being propagated in a sure and true way.

These people were anxious to learn as much as they could during their short stay in Babaji's midst. They listened and watched as he ministered to the Indian people's ails, healing with the use of his own Himalayan herbal remedies as well as spiritual healing. His healing was simple. He used the Name of God in all things. He took prayers from the Koran and was always sure of a right outcome in his healing work.

Babaji's hospitality to all visitors was total. He saw to the welfare of his foreign visitors who were fed the living food, cooked on an open fire, giving the food the energy of the sun through the living flame of the wood. He used only good quality grains and vegetables and knew where his supplies came from, grown naturally with no artificial growing aids of man's making.

The Westerners arrived at the ashram dressed and groomed to honour Babaji. Their glowing faces waited for his first appearance of the day. As he came through from his private quarters into the common area of the ashram, his people rose up as one and bent down to touch his feet. He beamed his smile across the sea of faces and one by one the devotees were led towards him with their individual requirements of their Babaji. The Westerners were patient and waited their turn. They knew Babaji's attention would be total and all elements of the lesson would be covered by the end of the afternoon, for review the following day.

The time arrived and they were directed into the drawing room where all praying, meditation and yoga was practised. They seated themselves in the semi-lotus position, though some were more used to it than others. The important factor was to have a straight and upright back, Babaji told them.

"A bent back does not aid the flow of energy," he said as he sat on the raised settee before his students, in the full lotus position. "Now, watch me. The breath is drawn up from the mooladhara (base) chakra, up the spine, until it reaches the throat chakra. As you breath in, you say, 'Who am I?' and then hold the breath, locked at the throat. This is the key," he said and pointed to the soft skin at the base of his throat.

"The breath is to be held for a short time whilst your eyes turn upwards to look at the third eye location in your brow. Feel the energy move up into the pineal. It will expand

and take you into the realms of higher consciousness. Then push the breath back down the front, pushing the energy down from the top of the head, through each of the five chakras from the throat to the mooladhara. As you breath out you say 'So I am.' As you breath in, you raise your arms, like so, like the wings of a swan, and say, 'Who am I?' and as you breath out you fold your arms back in, covering the heart chakra with your hands. It is such a beautiful exercise and it is so important that you know who you are. Eventually, you will hear the Song of God inside you and you will know the secret of who you are."

Babaji was smiling before his followers, whose eyes beheld the Master of kriya yoga demonstrate this seemingly simple process. They did not anticipate the power of the kriyas, however, and when they made their first attempts at controlling their breath in the way that Babaji had taught, some were immediately transported into a release of congested energies at different chakra points, depending on their individual issues. They would try and try again until the in and out breathing became easier and more relaxed. The swan-like movement of the arms became like a real feeling of a bird in flight. 'Who am I?...So I am...Who am I?...So I am.'

"Ah, my children, I see you are beginning to master the swan kriya . Practise this for a minimum of 15 to 20 minutes each day and soon you will feel the breath energising all parts of the body. The fire within you will be ignited and the Song of God will be with you, cleansing and healing, inside and out. Do the kriyas each day and you will travel your path to eternity. Stoke you fires and take your first steps to freedom."

He then left the room, leaving the newcomers to continue their breathing practice under the watchful eye of the Divine Mother.

The Best Things in Life

The mountains shone back at Babaji as he surveyed the scene before him. He never ceased to be calmed by their stoic, majestic countenance. They were his partners in his mission to give the Righteous Path to the people with listening ears. Those who could not hear his cry from the mountain would be salvaged somehow, but everything was in the right way of things for the moment. God's work was being honoured by all who came to Babaji for words of wisdom and direction.

The sun was reflecting with all its might the picture of abundance which Mother Earth held in her womb. She had everything man required. The best things in life were free. It was the attention of man which was to be sharpened if he were to succeed in living a life of ease, honouring his Creator, the All Loving, Living, One God of Ultimate Power and Eternity. If only man could grasp the meaning of life, he would surely require nothing but the air that he breathes, the Breath of God.

The Saviour was due to return shortly. He had protected mankind for a full 2000 years in accordance with his Seal of the Messiah. Babaji knew these to be the End of Days and it was of the utmost importance that the land was made as clear as possible for his brother, Jesus, to return as Punisher. God's Will was moving onwards and Mother Earth was being made ready for her place in the Story of Armageddon. This time she would be flattened.

Babaji's thoughts and prayers continued to build upon the requirements of Mother Earth as time was passing ever quicker towards the End of Days. He performed his morning ritual cleansing as he prepared for his next discourse. He knew it might disconcert even some of the more 'level-headed' of his devotees, but the message had to be given, otherwise they would not comprehend the impunity of their own matters. They needed to be prepared for their meeting with the Eternal and Most Loving God. Babaji decided to visit the ash tree at the front of the ashram.

A rug would be placed at the foot of the tree today, where his people could sit in comfort as he delivered his message to them. There would be special prashad distributed among them, as he felt the day to be special, too. Babaji sought out the cook in the outside wood-burning cookhouse and gave instruction on the exact manner he wanted the food preparing; the different quantities of appropriate spices and the method to be used for the best results. He enjoyed the science of food and took an active role in the provision of the daily prashad for all visitors to the ashram. His knowledge as a doctor and herbalist ensured that all food was provided with optimum care for the highest good of all. He cared greatly for the welfare of his flock.

He then made his way down to the ash tree, his long, shoulder-length hair gave him the sphinx-like look of a great master which, indeed, he was. He always told the story of the prophet, Joseph, who was Akhenaton, Pharaoh of Egypt. His crowing head-piece was the same as the widely known picture of Babaji. There were lessons to be given on the lineage of man and his origins when the next opportunity presented itself. In the meantime, the pressing facts of the third birth of man was to be related to the people that day.

He approached the ash tree with a reverence due to his Maker, the Lord God. He greeted the tree with the love of all Mother Nature's creation, and he was truly accorded with a matching love from the tree itself. It was one of the best things in life that never failed to happen, the reciprocation of unconditional love of life. The ash tree was of fine heart and would support the occasion this day. It was not long before there were many eyes upon Babaji and a gathered crowd was awaiting his words.

"The End of Days in looming ever nearer," he began, "due to the wrong actions of man. As he continues down his dead-end road to ruin with his weapons of mass destruction and self-ego worshipping, the fine balance of this earth's ecology is unable to sustain the pillage of her resources much longer. We have taken the same course as other greater civilisations and this time the earth will be flattened. The earth will be made as paper by the angels of mercy, who watch all manner of actions taken by the inhabitants of our living planet, Mother Earth. They see each travesty of mankind's blind ego's doing and making. They are the angels of mercy, here to see that we are kept in order, moving towards our Creator and Benefactor, in preparation for the resurrection. They are our support in the divine order of all that is. They will only be of assistance when asked, and man has still to learn to work with these wondrous beings of light of God's creation." Babaji hardly stopped for breath as he pressed on with the facts of man's third birth.

"The resurrection of the earth's population is due shortly. This will be our third birth and the Day of Reckoning, when all of mankind will be made to be transparent about his deeds of good and bad. Each person's Book of Life will be opened and read, page by page, and according to each individual's efforts in making his way on the Eternal Path, his sins will be forgiven and witnessed by the 'made-easy' they walked alongside in their everyday life. Masters and mentors of all time will present their flocks, one by one, for salvation. Those who turned a blind eye to the right way of living will not be accompanied by such prophets and masters and, depending on the balance sheet of their karmas, will either ascend to heaven or descend to a hell appropriate to the extent of the gravity of their sins. All will be accounted for, my children."

The atmosphere of the crowd was uncertain as they gave their own personal thought to their misdemeanours, great and small. How would they fare when the Day of Reckoning arrived? What would be the outcome? Babaji could see what was turning around in their minds and offered solace.

"Do not worry, my children. I will be alongside you when you go before your Maker. The four great angels will be sitting on the Seat of God and I shall say to the Lord God, 'Forgive him his sins, Lord, for he has followed me on my path and bowed down before Thee in honour of Thy Name. I witness this man's conscious and unconscious sins and forgive him in Thy Name, Lord.' You will be the judge of your own misdemeanours and self-punishment will be yours. And you will take a third birth into the realms of goodness and mercy, where all people will love their neighbour, honour their parents and do no wrongful deed. The people will be at one with God and you will know great joy and happiness. Walk the path steadfastly and the benefits will be yours to eternity. Live a clean life and all will not be lost to you. The best things in life are free and you shall know the bliss of a life of freedom, when the End of Days moves the Will of God onwards and upwards. Be free, my seed of the future. Be free."

By now the ash tree had its essence enveloped around each person. All were given its gift through the Light of God, as He worked His wonders in the never ending circles of Mother Nature's store of vibrational healing. The ash tree is able to restore the faith in God that man has let go of. The strength of this particular tree would always recoup the balance of God's Nature into the wilting soul of the unbeliever.

"Come unto me," said the Lord Jesus. "The fields of succour are open to all who follow me. Open your hearts and minds to all things possible in the Way of the One Omniscient God. You shall be uplifted and know the bliss of His Eternal Presence."

The Initiator

The days passed by, one by one, and the western visitors came and went. More than one returned on a regular basis, each time working on new issues of their own but, more importantly, they came to learn. Once learnt, Babaji told them it was their duty to pass on their revelations to those who were lost in the rituals and traditions of their ancestors, or the dead gods and idols of man's modern day making. The lessons were given to them in bite-size chunks depending on where they were in their own game plan, but always they came away with thought-provoking stimuli of Babaji's inimitable teaching methods. He never minced his words, never fearing to contradict long-standing theological understanding wherever he knew it to be wrong. He had the most direct way of putting a point across, and if it did not match the lessons of the mainstream religions, it would quite often throw some of his devotees into disconcerting periods of inner searching and questioning.

"Can the facts be right that Babaji has given us? How can it be that the religions have got some revelations so wrong?" his devotees have asked themselves, with an uncomfortable feeling within their third chakra of willpower and inner knowing. They were put to the test straight away on the issue of trusting this Master and Guru. After all, he was holding himself responsible as witness to their Book of Life on their Day of Reckoning.

The truth is that he is a Maha Avatar and messenger of the Lord God. He has existed on Mother Earth in physical form continuously, to be the cry on the mountain for Jesus. His words are revealed to us from Jesus, who directs the facts through Babaji, who then translates into English or Hindi, depending on the mix and meld of the attending crowd. He switches from one language to another with an ease and intuitive knowledge of who needs to know what bit of information and when. His discourses can go on for seemingly endless periods of time, but he never falters in his work. His mission is to prepare people for the resurrection, when they will return once more to their Lord God. He says he does not care if he is believed or not. It does not matter if people choose to reject his revelations, but the ones who have ears for the truth, and walk, talk and breath the Righteous Path, will be given salvation. It does not matter if you are a Christian, Moslem, Jew or Hindu. He is not here to bring a new religion in this world or convert people. He just says you should be a good Christian or a good Hindu. Whichever walk of life you adhere to, his missive is to propagate the message of One-God worshipping, to worship only the One Living and Eternal God, in whichever form you see Him, but not to laud and magnify the dead gods and relics of man-made thinking and manufacture. This is the road to ruin in no uncertain terms.

This messenger of the One Omniscient, Eternal and Most Merciful God receives people from all over the world into his fold. He sees at once whether they are of right-thinking, and wastes little time on those who are not of a true nature, who are there maybe for material gain. When he sees a person of clean heart, he will start to work on their lessons immediately, always giving what is required at the exact right moment for them to be magnetised towards the Dharma, the Righteous Path. It may be that someone needs time to sit back and listen before he approaches them with a personal revelation, for their ears only, and this process can take any number of weeks, but the professional fisherman knows just when to hook his catch. The initiation is a right of passage afforded by this Master when an individual has made his mark, whether he be advanced in introspection or has arrived fresh from the halls of his ancestral worship. He initiates all who are of pure heart, whose desire is to find out who they are and to learn how to follow the Dharma.

These people are the chosen beings. Babaji is here to gather the chosen beings, who will help with the sifting out of the bad seed amongst the seed of God's creation. The Garden of God is ever evolving and the weeds of old stock need to be plucked out from the realms of this space on earth. The way to God-realisation is through the feeding of one's inner-self with the succour of the Heavenly Father and our dear Mother Earth. The Initiator is here to guide us.

The Importance of Living Food

The inner realms are full of highways and bye-ways, some of which can be blocked with unhealthy air and a foul way of feeding ourselves. The air becomes stale within us when it is not replenished with good clean air of right breathing. It is the same, of course, with the elements taken in by food.

Babaji considered it of the utmost importance that his people were taught the knowledge of the different energies and where they came from. Today was to be a day of such discourse, and he felt the aid of the flowers within the grounds of his ashram would hold his students in good reception whilst this information was absorbed into their systems. They needed to know the difference between the red and green energies with the multitude of cadences in between. The deep orange colour of the nasturtiums which grew in profusion around the ashram was perfect for fulfilment of his words today. Its healing properties included that of helping the digestion system, and at the same time improving the relationship with one part of the physical body with that of the more subtle regions of one's being. Indeed, the nasturtium was ideal for the occasion.

As usual, the area was cleaned and prepared by the servants at the ashram. It was always done with good intent and a loving movement. Babaji's followers slowly began to arrive, making themselves at home in the higher air of his mountain abode. They greeted each other with words of peace, in whichever language they spoke, and positioned themselves ready for their Babaji's presence amongst them. The sheer magnitude of his loving aura was sufficient to feed their own spiritual appetite.

They did not have to wait long this day and soon his smiling eyes were upon them, radiating the Love of the Lord God in powerful surges, in and amongst the crevices of the individual shades of need and inner cleansing. It was not that his devotees were lazy in their daily routine of inner and outer cleansing, but rather that their systems had become choked up with a culmination of issues, both mental and physical. The day was, indeed, ripe for the discourse of eating the living food.

"As Salam a lakum, my children. May God's Will Be Done this day. You are all of good spirit and the sunshine is recharging your batteries in the beautiful clean air of my ashram. Let us now take this opportunity of thanking our Creator for the abundance of life and our blessings thus received. He is the All Merciful and Giving Lord God and we bow down in honour of His gifts this day. The flowers are smiling towards their Maker and the birds are singing the Lord's Song of Life. The positive energy of all of Mother Nature surrounds us. Breathe in deeply her life-force, the blessings of our Lord God." The gathering did as they were bid and Babaji once more breathed in the Almighty's life supporting Breath of God.

"Now, I shall give you the Salve of God, the benefit of the alive food from which to take the energy of the sun and Mother Earth, herself. There are many kinds of food energy sources and if you are to fair well, consider it important to pay attention to which energy source it is that your body requires at any one time. The sources are profound and are gifts to be honoured. Always give thanks to the Lord God after taking the fruits of His making. The nearer to Mother Earth your food source is, the cleaner and more alive will be the life-force within it. The further away the food is from its original source, by way of man's manufacture, the less energy it will have to sustain your minds and bodies. Remember, you are feeding your mind, body and spirit when partaking of God's Food.

"The green energy is the energy from plants and trees. This is the purest form of food from which you are able to ingest the sun energy directly. The plant has processed the sun rays upon its foliage through photosynthesis and retained all its positive energies. When you eat the plant, all the time giving thanks to your Lord God, the energy will be changed into living protein of your own. You will radiate the positive attributes of that plant out into the universe for all to benefit from. The plant also draws in the goodness of Mother Earth through its roots. The elements of the particular region of dear Mother Earth are integrated into the plant's attributes, including the metals and minerals of her soil. All these are made by the combined alchemy of the sun and Mother Earth, so that mankind is sustained. This is the green energy of the flora and fauna, which grows in great numbers of species all over the land from high up in the mountains to the low plains of the meandering rivers. The water energy, too, is taken into the life-force of the plants, the energy of movement, not of a rigid nature. Take heed of all manner of clues which are there to show you that which is best for your own particular needs of the day: the lie of the land, the moon phases, too, should be considered but, most importantly, make your choice of foods to be the living food of the Almighty and Most Beneficent God. He is the Maker of all things and you shall always be provided for.

"The green energy can also make its way to you by the positive food chain of God's fine creatures which have been provided to man for his subsistence. These animals are of the red energy, but they feed from the clean plants and vegetation of the land, converting the green energy into red energy, protein. Beware of the source of the red energy. Take care that you know from where the cow or goat has fed before drinking its milk. If the animal has been fed the dead energy source of man's making then do not partake of it. Ensure that the milk is from a beast which has been fed the clean fodder of the land and herbs from the high hills, each with their own healing properties. It is of great benefit to you when the mountain goats eat from the steep slopes of the terrain where you are unable to climb. By drinking its milk you are energised by the positive energy of the mountain tops, the clean air of the winds, without pollution from man's machinery and refuse."

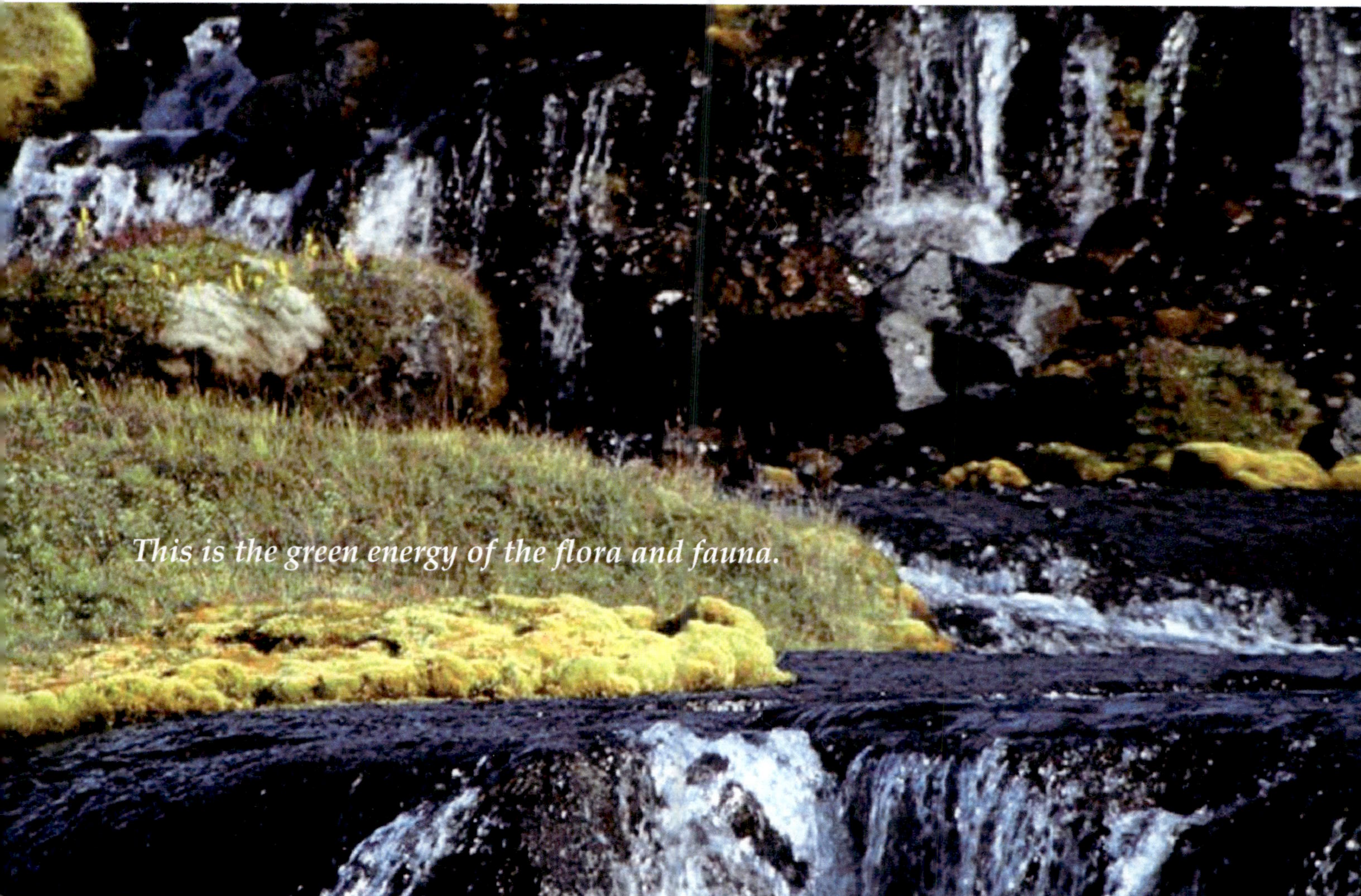
This is the green energy of the flora and fauna.

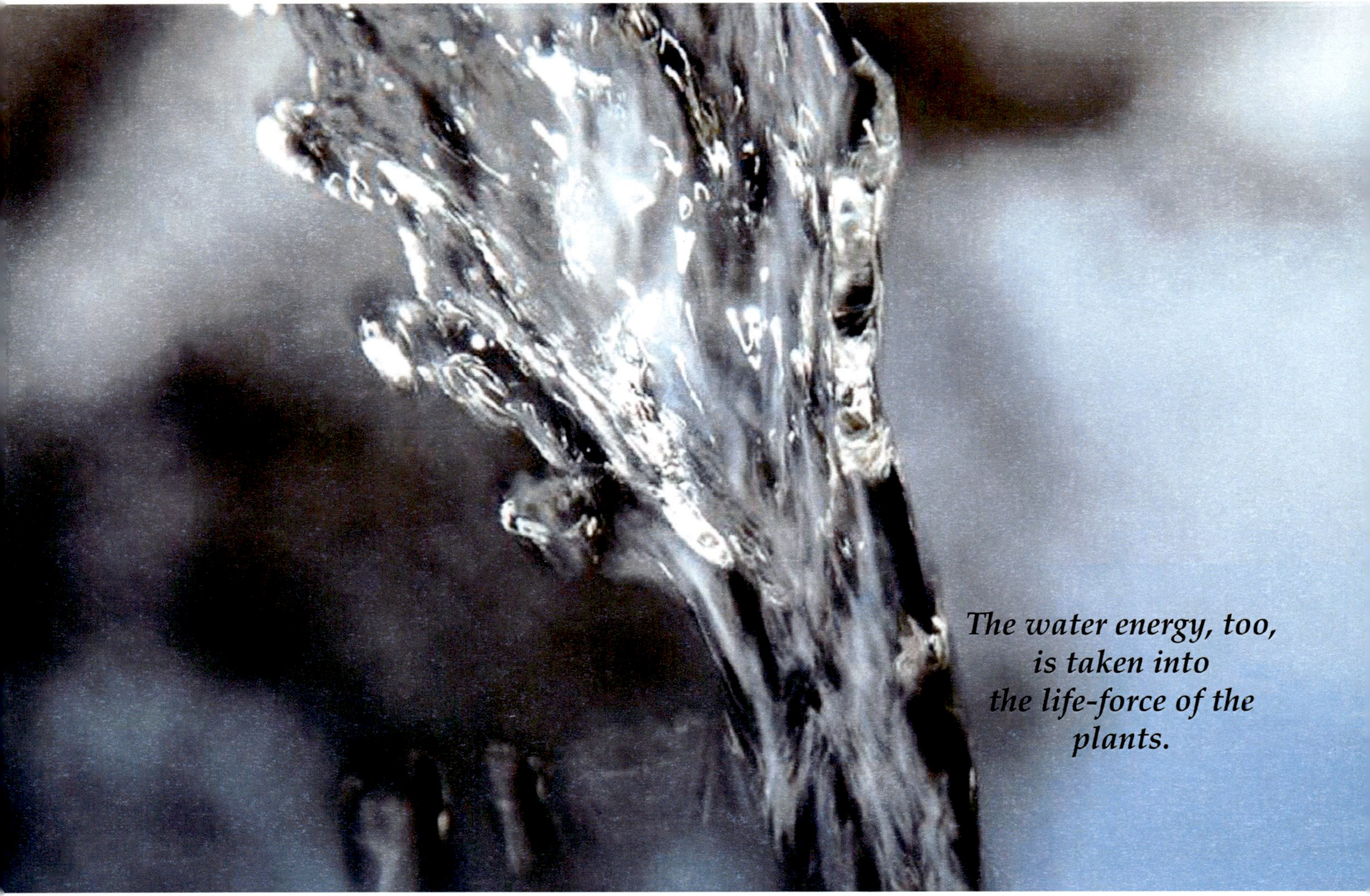

The water energy, too,
is taken into
the life-force of the
plants.

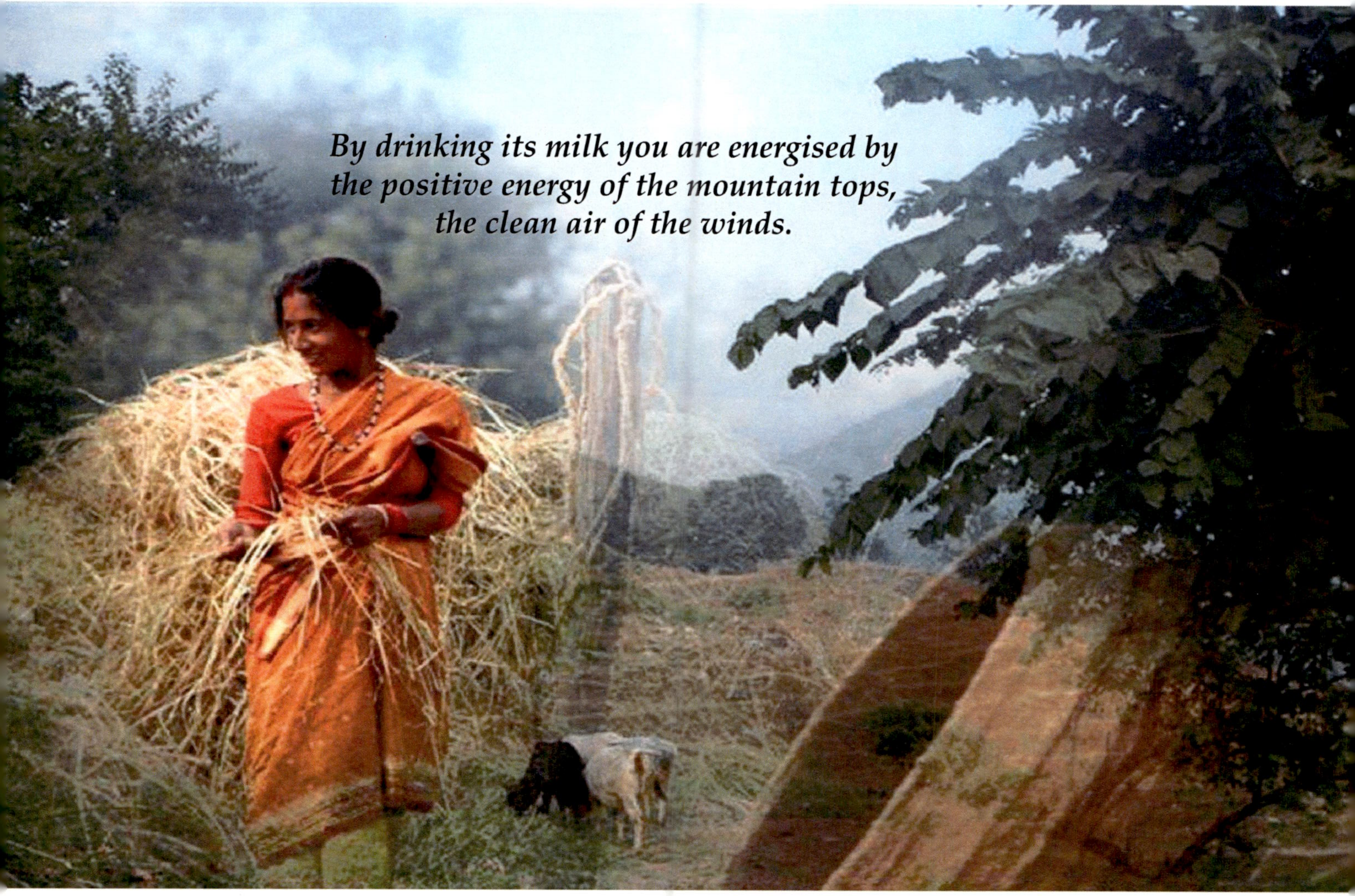
By drinking its milk you are energised by
the positive energy of the mountain tops,
the clean air of the winds.

They would work together at creating cleaner and alive food.

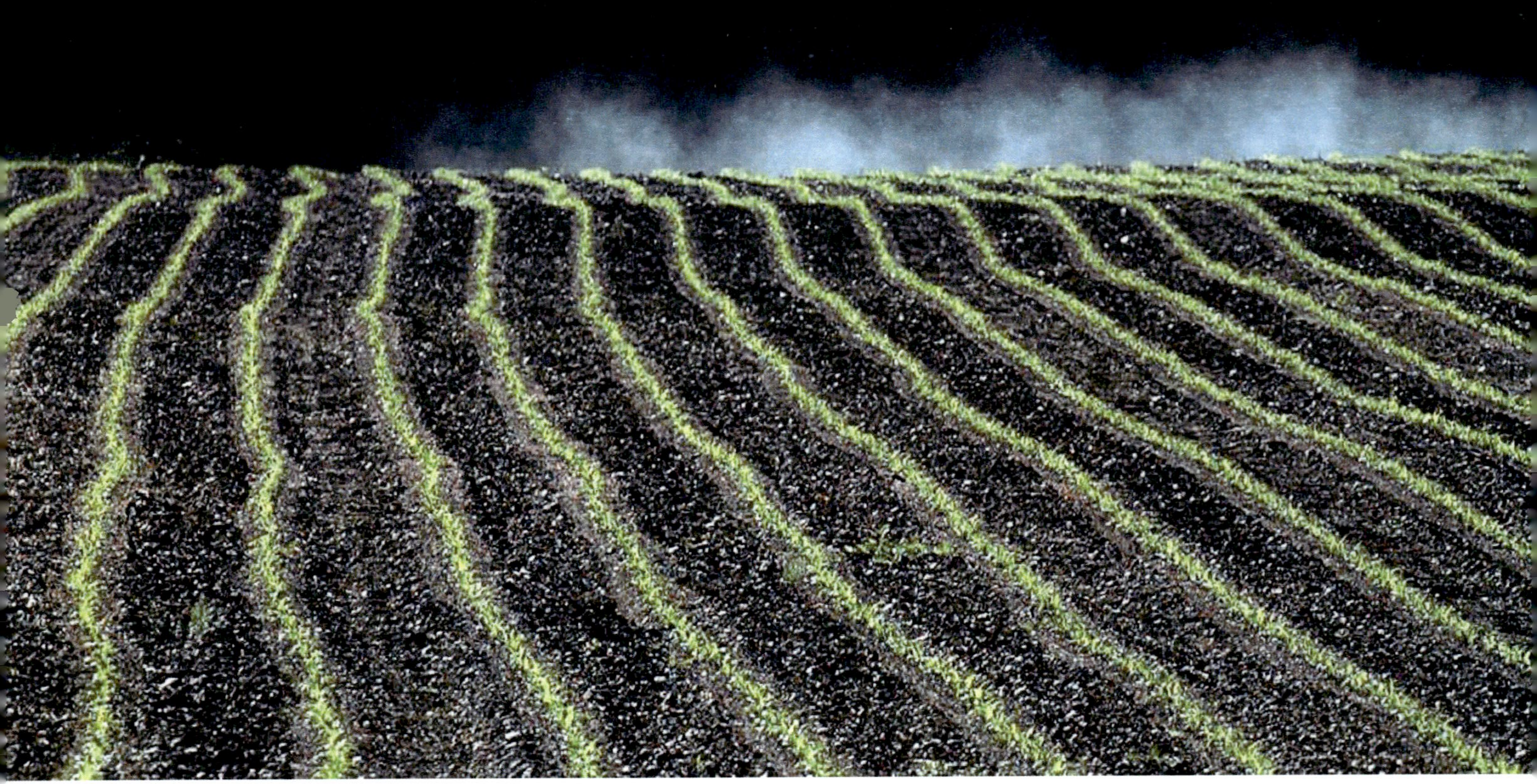

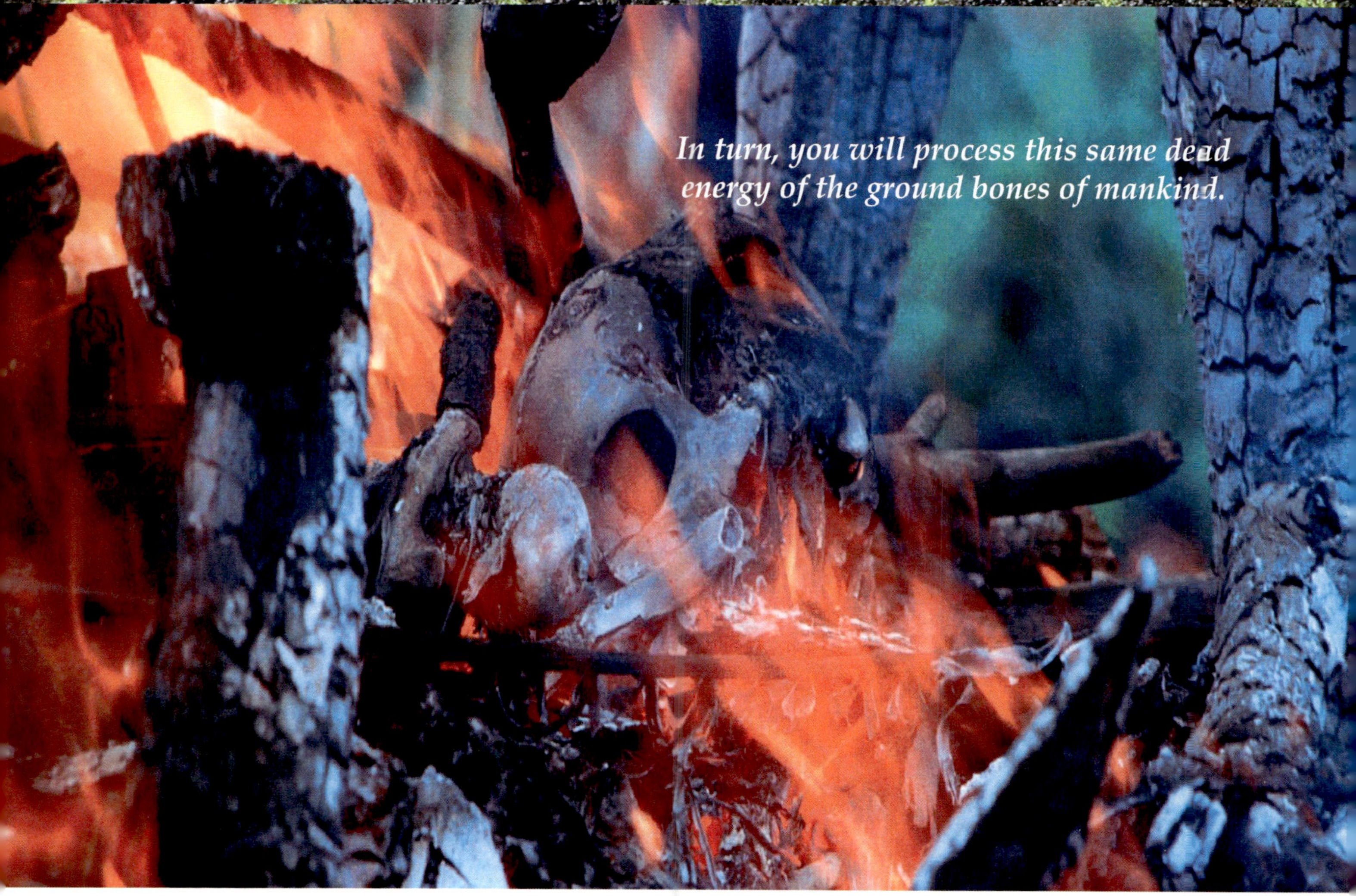

In turn, you will process this same dead energy of the ground bones of mankind.

The crowd all nodded in agreement with Babaji's words. They were beginning to understand the concept of what he was saying. They were of accord and would do their utmost to live as pure a lifestyle as possible within the realms of civilisation. They would work together at creating cleaner and alive food from their own gardens and market places. It was important that this living food was available to all in the community. A mother's breast milk was only as good as she, herself, had eaten and her baby requires the alive food, too. Babaji continued.

"It is not always possible to be a good vegetarian when considering the land on which one lives. It may be that the land is poor agriculturally. There may be extreme weather systems in the region or continent, for example, the desert or ice caps of the north and south poles. In these instances it is permissible for man to eat the flesh of animals, such as cows and sheep, those beasts of cloven-hoof, who chew the grass. Or, if you live by the ocean, then to eat the seafood is acceptable. Of course, the energy is the red energy that is being ingested from the animal, and seafood is of the white energy. Whatever you do, eat for God Who will accept that the animals and sea creatures have sacrificed their own lives in honour of that of your own. Thank the Lord for His Loving Compassion as you eat the dead meat or fish. Whenever you have the need to eat such food, pay tribute to the beast and ensure that its life has been a life of ease. Ensure, too, that it has eaten the alive food of Mother Earth's provision rather than the dead relics of man's making, such as the ground bones of man, himself, and other chemical fodders. There is no energy in such food and it will be processed as dead energy by the animal itself. In turn, you will process this same dead energy of the ground bones of mankind. Avoid the dense vibration of such food which will dullen your own vibrational existence. It is best to be good vegetarians, eating the food of a light and vibrant nature, in accordance with the seasons of Mother Earth.

"Yet another form of conversion of the green energy is by insects. Insects are of the yellow energy. For example, bees collect the pollen of the blossom and convert it into honey, one of nature's most wondrous nectars fit for human consumption. As with the example of the mountain goat eating different herbs on the high hills, so, too, do the bees collect from the infinite variety of flowers and blossoms. Try to ensure that your choice of honey is as pure as possible, taking consideration of its source. Again, it is all too easy to purchase honey which has been chemically treated by man and his manufacturing processes for a longer shelf-life in our shops. These methods introduce an artificial element to the honey or, indeed, to many other manufactured foodstuffs.

"So, my children, the food that you eat makes you the person that you are, and if you fall into bad habits of eating the hog meat, the snake meat or the dog, then you will surely sink into unrighteous living. The earth provides everything that mankind requires if he lives according to the law of nature, God's Law. Live for the welfare of the Creation of God. Live in universal brotherhood. This means not killing man or beast. It means caring for each other as you would yourself. Be charitable to all living things, including the plants and trees. Honour their existence alongside that of your own."

The knowledge that Babaji was handing over to his disciples was of the highest importance. It enveloped the whole essence of the meaning of life. The Laws of God were the key to man's success in loving and living the Righteous Path. All elements of mankind's lessons were contained within the limits of His Commandments. Mankind was, indeed, fortunate to have the mission of Babaji to uphold these laws, to remind him of the Almighty God's wish that man followed the way back to Him in all things that he did. Man was here on Mother Earth to know Him and be with Him. Pure living was the highest accolade to the Almighty Creator. He will surely smile down upon those who strive for a clean lifestyle, inside and out, who master the art of living.

Babaji considered the final part of the day's message to his people about the different energies of their food sources: how to prepare the food to its optimum benefit for consumption. He stood before them and pointed towards the outside cookhouse of his ashram, as smoke gently bellowed out from the open windows in preparation of the evening prashad, Babaji's offering to all visitors. The fire was being ignited by the cook and the flames would soon be at the correct temperament for cooking the grain and vegetables.

"See how I choose the living source of energy on which to cook our food. This energy source is equally as important as the choice of living food with which to sustain our bodies. The fire has an alive element, that of the sun. When the wood was alive as a branch of a tree, it took in all the strength of the sun, and absorbed the energy into its fibres. You may think that the wood is dead, but it still contains the life-force of the sun as well as that of Mother Earth, when she sustained the tree as it grew. The process of photosynthesis was the kriya of the tree's existence, the breath of life, and when we burn the wood to cook our food, positive energy comes out in the form of a living frame. We get the benefit of its power when we sit before the fire as we cook, as well as within the food we eat. The tree's life-force is given to you and it should be honoured for its gifts. Thank the Lord God for His every gift as the day starts, and send out the message of His Song within you into the many schools of life on this earth: the art of living."

There was more to tell about the use of green energy within the wider context of the art of living, but his disciples had had sufficient information to mentally digest for the moment. The mountain mists were rolling down the valley, enveloping the land and tree tops. The air had become chilly and people were wrapping themselves up with their shawls. Babaji noted the fabric of their clothes and felt it appropriate to talk about the green energy and the clothes they adorn themselves with. This was to be the subject of his next lesson in the art of living.

"As Salam a lakum, my children. Be at peace. The night is drawing in and you have homes to return to. Keep the art of living at the centre of your thoughts these next days and observe what changes you can make in your consciousness towards the essence of being a good human being. The time is nigh that all communities make severe adjustment to the way people interact and live according to the Law of God, the Ten Commandments, the law of nature. I will talk more on the art of living in order to clarify some of the misinterpretations of mankind of what is good and righteous living and what is dead living, the lifestyle of the dead beings," Babaji concluded.

When the last of the people had dispersed, Babaji went into his inner domain, all the time communing with his Beloved Creator and Eternal God. He would spend the next minutes in meditation to replenish his life's fire within. It was the end of the day and he, too, enjoyed relaxing with his family and close friends. It was good to maintain a balance of work and relaxation, but the kriyas were always there to assist when energy levels were low after a long day's work. Life was truly good.

Further Considerations of The Green Energy

The air of the day was fresh and Babaji breathed in deep. He felt that time was in the green phase of things. The planet was adjusting her plasma and this meant that its inhabitants would experience discomfort, some more severely than others, depending on their mode of life. It was necessary for Mother Earth to make her movements, otherwise she would not withstand the imbalance that man had created upon her and within her. The oceans, too, would make their discomfort felt and their forces would cleanse the areas of density that were becoming too much to bear. It was the law of nature, the Law of Cause and Effect. Man knows this law quite clearly but remains ignorant as to how it works in practise. Babaji would continue his mission to make those people aware of their actions and non-actions, who would spread the Word of God out to others who would otherwise not hear. God was available to all earth's populations, but some were totally in the dark. They would perish if the Word were not broadcast to them. Babaji would initiate those who were of the positive vibration of Godly-consciousness. It would be a testing time for them, but he surrendered them to the Will of God and God's Will Be Done.

Babaji was giving further consideration of the green energy and how he might persuade his disciples to pay heed to his words of advice. He decided to wander down to the lake and find a good place to give his message. The trees would be a good shield and enhancer of his work as everyone sat beneath the vibrations of the pure greenness of their nature. The lake, too, would reflect the light of the sun towards the people's receptive systems of vibrational energy. The water energy would loosen up the resistance of any rigid mindset, ingrained by the indoctrination from birth of mankind's life-flow, rather than that of natural living. Oh, how mankind made life difficult for himself by making such laws that seemingly were for the benefit of a structured civilisation. In fact, it was the case that the only people to benefit from this lifestyle were the ones who had set themselves up as leaders, the lords and gods of man, himself, who enjoyed the ill-gotten gains of a selfish, deviated path to ruin. The Law of God was immovable. The truth always comes out and the energy adjusts accordingly.

The thoughts and prayers of Babaji continued, ever-flowing for the love of his people inspite of their misguided ways. Some were more open in their way of thinking and it would be these devotees he would ensure received his message on green energy. His repetitive words always made their mark and he never tired of speaking the truth. He settled beneath a beautiful larch tree, which would help with the interpretation of God's Word into the limited thinking of man's capabilities. The green energy of this tree was the most beneficial for his words to sink into the distorted systems of his people, due to wrong living. This was how wrong living blocked the flow of God's Breath, and it was a prime example of why man had to alter his existence, in order to feel God to his maximum ability.

His devotees soon got word that their Master was waiting for them by the lake under the larch trees. They wondered why he had chosen to deliver his discourse in this space, but did not question its benefits. They knew Babaji had their utmost welfare at heart and trusted him implicitly.

"As Salam a lakum, my children. It is good that you were able to find me here. The air is good and the tree and water energy is perfect. Listen to the birds calling out God's Name. They are excellent at showing us where the finest energies are. So, we are here.

"Feel the benefit of the surrounding trees as you listen to my words today. The green energy is around us even as we learn about its positive properties. We should always live in the flow of nature in every task that we do. The provision of Mother Earth's treasure trove is abundant and we lack for nothing. God has created everything we need for a life of ease on our path towards Him. We are the lucky ones who are able to appreciate the plates of food before us. The green energy is the most beneficial energy and it is available in a multitude of forms. We have the trees, shrubs, plants and flowers around us, each with their unique healing properties. We do not need to know with precision what it is that they do. We only need to follow our body's requirements of the moment and be amongst the abundance of nature's gifts. As I said only yesterday, we can eat the energy of our plants, and cook with the energy of our trees as they diminish in their living form. Using wood energy from different trees will also give off the power of their unique flames.

"We should also give consideration to the clothes we put on our backs. Think about the different energies of the fabrics we wear. The green energy of plants is made up of natural fibres. The structure of their DNA is within the cellulose of their life form. By taking this fibre, which continues to exist as a living thing even after it has been plucked from its original life form, we can use the woven form of cotton and make our clothes with the material which is of the highest vibrational benefit. This is the green energy I am talking about and instruct you to use."

His devotees looked around at the various forms of fabric they were wearing amongst themselves. Some had already chosen the natural materials, but some were wearing the cloth of man's manufacture, or a mixture of both.

"Beware of the fabrics you see in the stores. Not all are what they seem. Man has taken the natural fibres and interwoven them with the dead fibres made of nylon, the dead energy of ancient relics, oil. This fibre is dangerous to man as it is full of negative energy, static electricity, which attracts the negative energy around you and your body. Be astute with your purchases of clothing. Be with the flow of nature's provision.

The air that we breath is the blue energy of the earth's atmosphere,
the sky, the Divine Father...the sea reflects the blue.

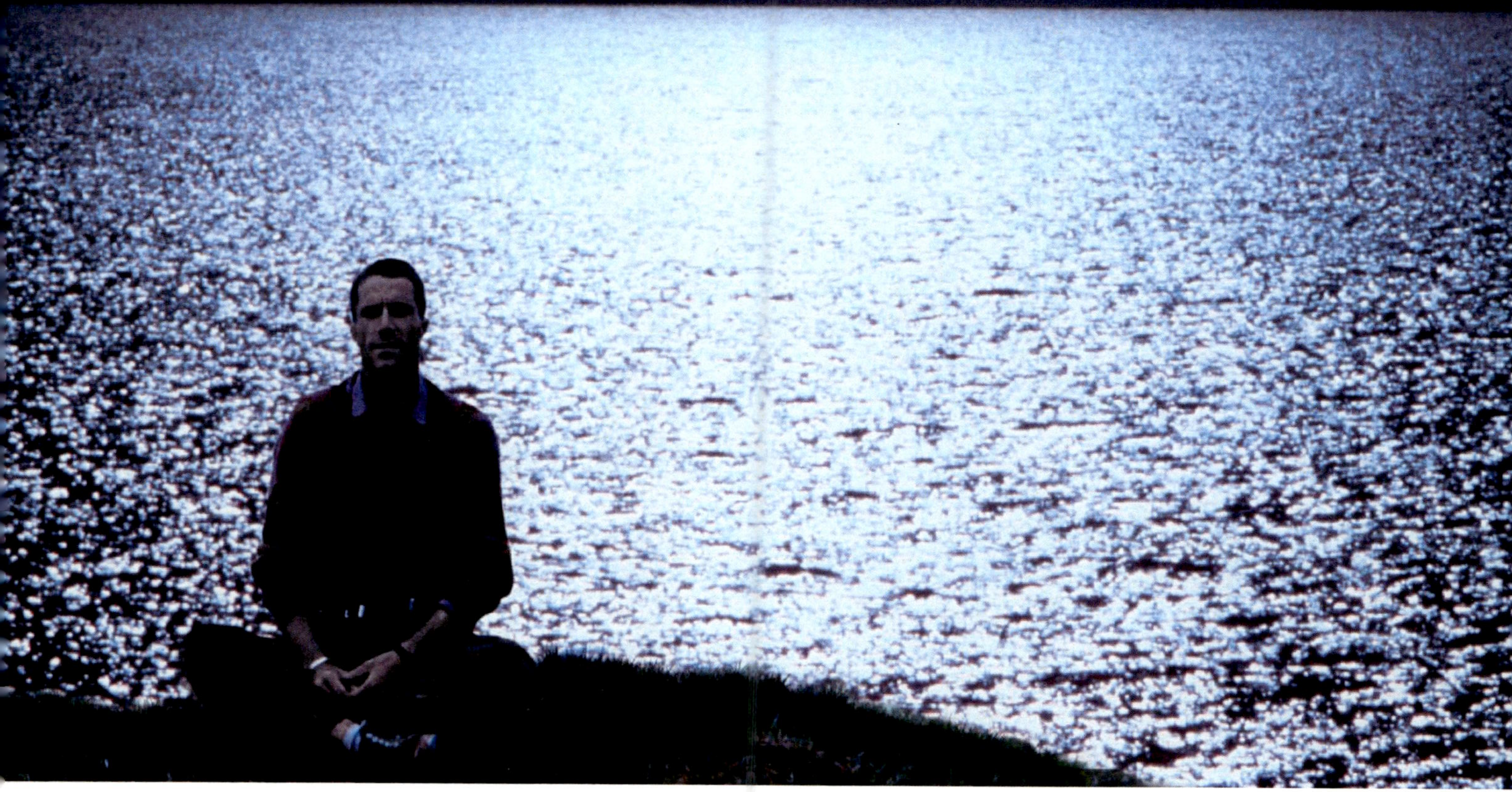

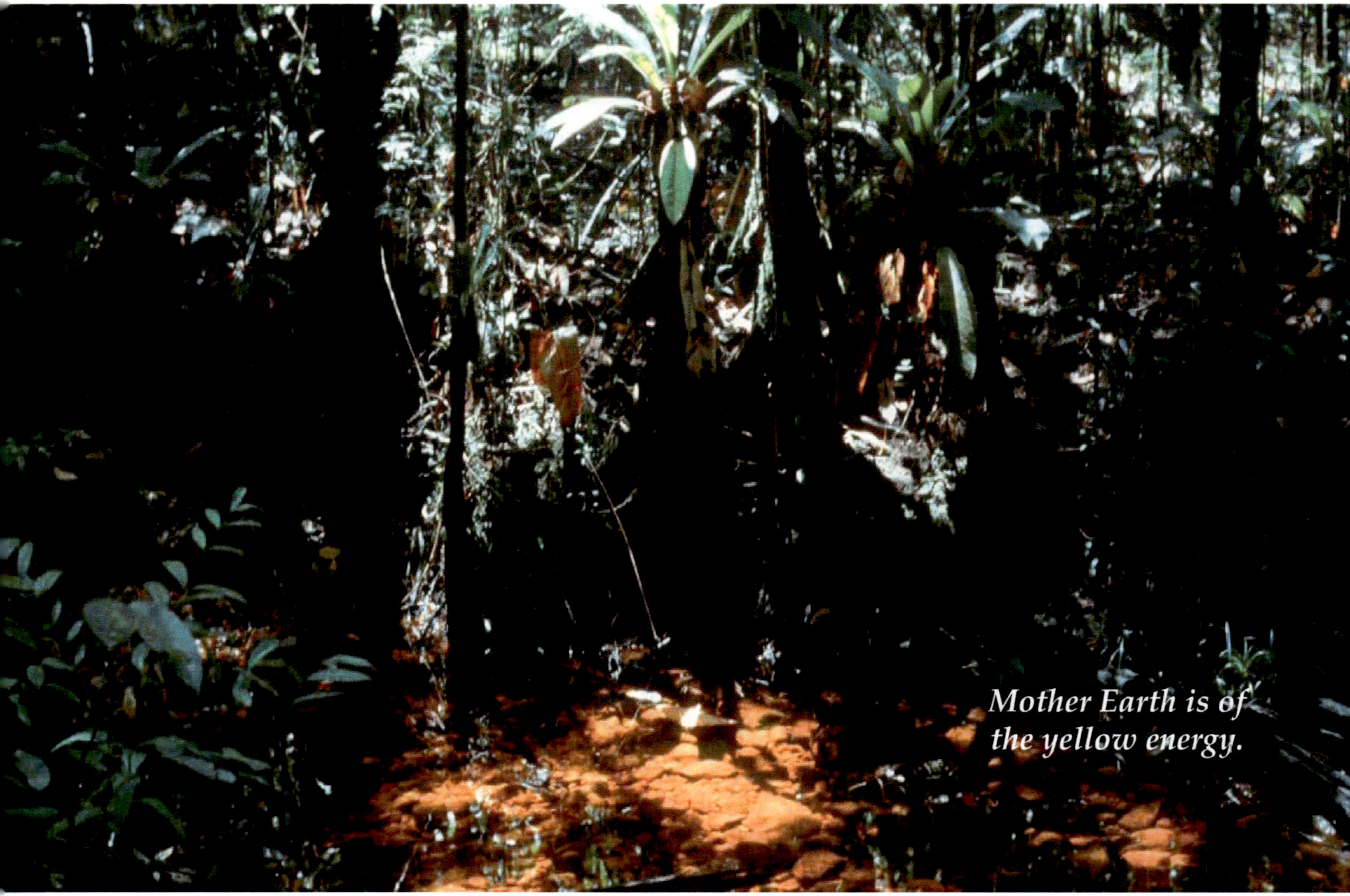

Mother Earth is of the yellow energy.

"We can go a step further, as Mother Nature converts the green energy into other proteins for us to use. As man has acquired the knowledge of weaving these natural materials, he has been able to utilise the product of the silkworm, insects of the yellow energy, and they convert the green protein into their yellow protein when they munch at the leaves and foliage of the plants. The silkworm converts the energy into the finest of threads with which they form their cocoons for transformation of their living forms. These threads are trillions and trillions of kilometers long and are hollow inside. They are a living fibre, like our own hair, and the Chinese have mastered the art of weaving this minute thread into cloth for us to wear. This is an excellent media that keeps us warm in the winter months and cool in the summer heat. This is the yellow energy.

"The green energy is also converted to the red energy by animals such as sheep, alpaca and such like. We take the fleece of a sheep and it is woven into sheets of fabric, or we can knit the thread into garments. This, also, is of a positive nature and can be utlised. However, again, beware of the mixed fibres that are interwoven with the natural stuff. Again, I tell you it is dangerous.

"Keep away from the chemical imitations and dye stuffs which are used in the modern fabrics. Man uses the metallic elements of the plants' DNA which are treated chemically, causing shinier and brighter colours, but they are totally artificial and are not conducive with the well-being of the human being. The electro-magnetic fields which are created in the fibres do not work alongside our own natural electro-magnetic field and thus negative energy is created. It is anti-nature. Use fabrics which have been treated according to nature, using natural dye stuffs of plants and trees. Then you will flow freely and easily in the way of nature's structure. In turn, you will give off the positive energy affecting those around you in a positive manner. It is nature's way and you are part of nature's patterned tapestry of life.

"Take full advantage of all things given by the Grace of God. The green energy is just one example of the infinite forms of positive matter which the Almighty God has created in this world. Everything is made up of some form of protein; strands upon strands of fibrous matter, some green, some red, some yellow, some white and there are any number of other types of matter with which our lives and environment around us has been manifested.

The air that we breath is the blue energy of the earth's atmosphere, the sky, the Divine Father. This blue energy colours our sky, and the sea reflects the blue. Mother Earth is of the yellow energy, and together the Divine Father (blue) and the Divine Mother (yellow) make the green energy.

"So, we are constructed with the five elements of earth, air, fire, water and ether, or cosmic dust of the Divine Father. These are the five elements which form the fibrous matter and from which everything is knitted together.

"If we live according to nature's law, God's Law, we will naturally flow in the direction of the Lord God. It is the way of things, and it is the way things were always intended to be by our Eternal, Living Lord God."

Babaji's words came to and end. His audience had been appreciative of his discourse and thanked him, touching his feet as they took their leave. As they did so, he gave each person a blessing by blowing his fiery breath on to their heads down to their base chakras. It was a loving gesture of a master to his students as they resolved to tap into all aspects of nature's abundant store. Surely there was no need of the artificial means of man. There was sufficient for all from Mother Earth's pantry and storerooms of cottons, silks, woollens and the like.

"Praise be to the Most Generous and Benevolent Lord God," chanted one old devotee as he stepped out on to the lake-side path, the evening air just beginning to chill. Babaji echoed the old man's thanks to the Almighty. The air seemed to stand still and had a tangible feel to it as the angels added their blessings to the cocktail of love and compassion of the Divine Mother and Divine Father that day.

The Story of Man's Heritage

From time to time God sends to man His messengers, prophets and rasools, to help him with his progress towards the Creator. These 'made-easies' come in the form of man, but are not born through the process of the blessing of Mother Earth and the Divine Father. They are born by the Grace of God, by His Word, the stories of whom are contained in the holy scriptures of the Holy Bible, Koran, Bhagavad Gita and the Scrolls. All stories have a great similarity in the content of their message, but the main players of the history of man have different names.

In his small room at the ashram, Babaji knew that there were facts in the holy scriptures which were distorted somewhat, either by genuine misunderstanding of the Word of God, or through the desire of man to create his own laws and religion for the benefit of himself. Babaji knew the truth and ensured that he regularly put across the message of God's Eternal Truth. It was his mission and he was passionate about the truth. He would remind his people today of the origins of man and his birthright. He took down the ancient Holy Bible from his high shelf and opened it at the Book of Genesis. The light began to filter into his room and the first of the day's blessings was upon him. Soon the people would arrive in anticipation of his blessings. The day would be fruitful, indeed.

The angels gathered together lifting the atmosphere an octave or two as Babaji's devotees arrived in ones and twos, all in right spirit for the day's agenda. The birds also sang in full accolade of the blessing of the day, and the trees and plants, too, waved their leaves and blooms with the whispering of God's Breath. Babaji made his entrance, beaming his radiant, loving smile to all.

"As Salam a lakum. Let us quickly settle to the day's work, my children." There were small children running and playing in and amongst the gathered people. The mix of the playful energies of the young ones created a light-heartedness in the air which would help when the lesson

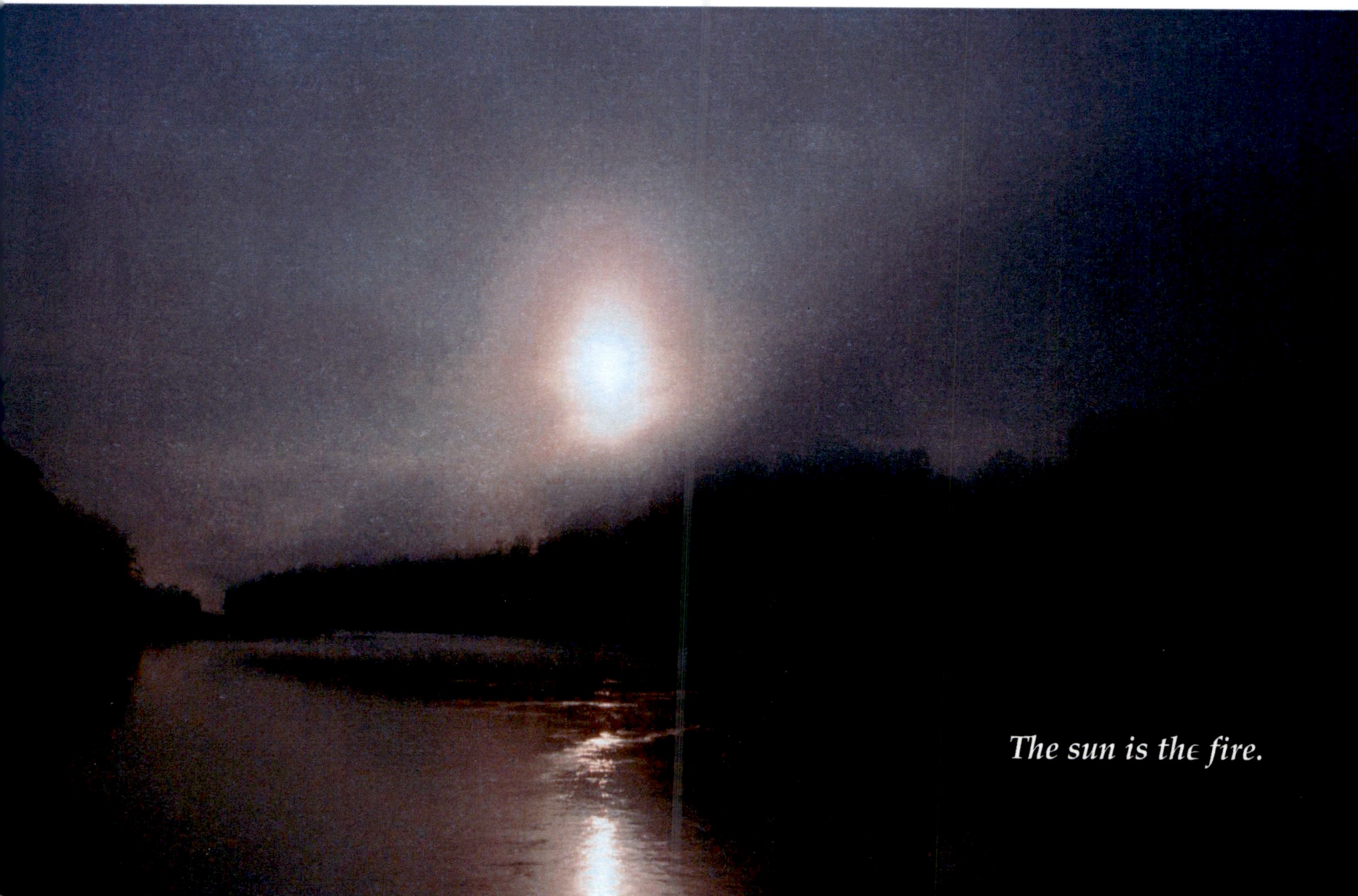

The sun is the fire.

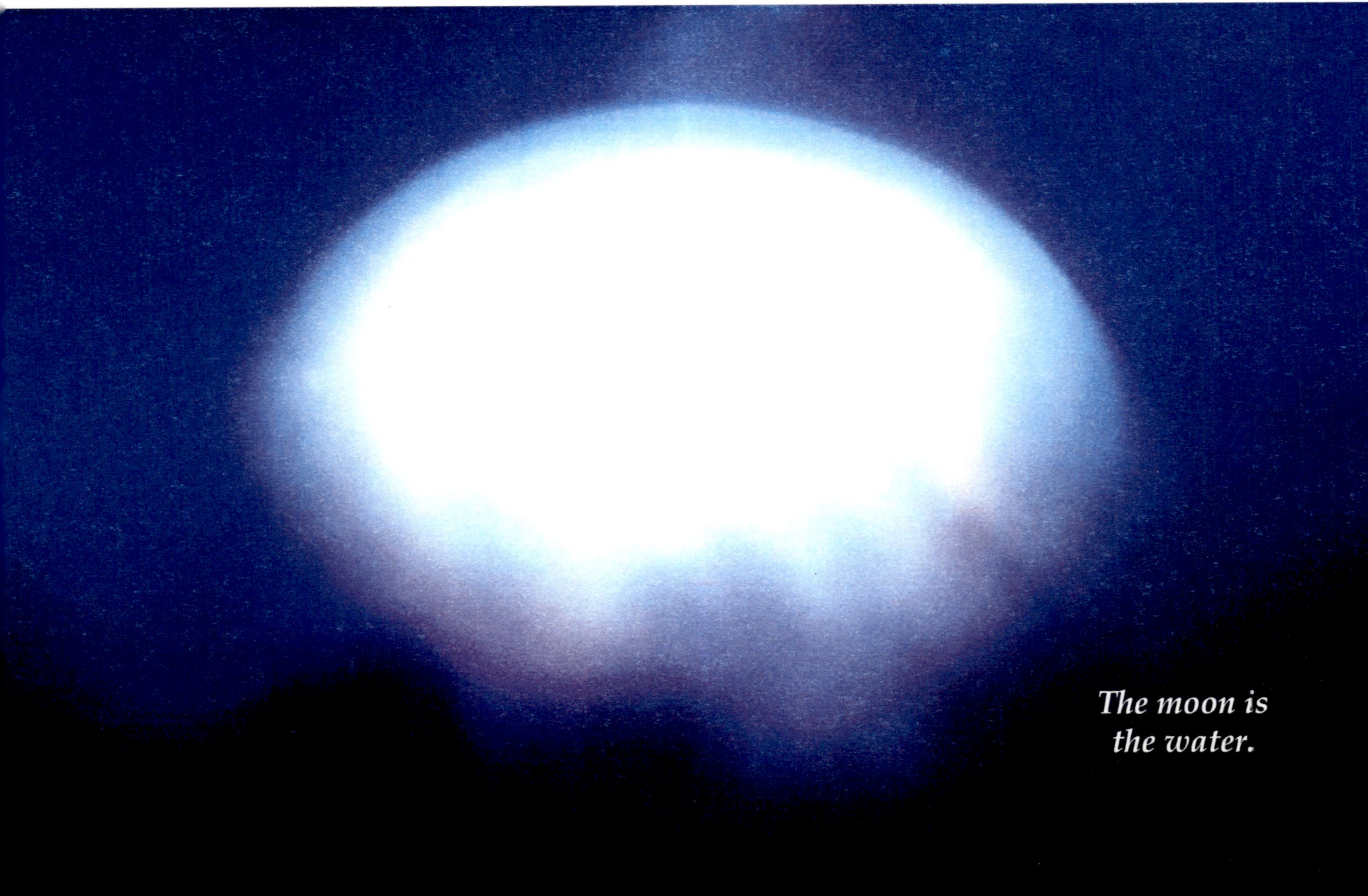
The moon is
the water.

got into full flow. Babaji loved the presence of his grandchildren, the children of his children, and gave great hugs and kisses to the receptive innocence of the youth.

"We are made by the blessing of the Divine Father and the Divine Mother. We are of the sun and the moon. The sun is the fire and the moon is the water, which is the media of our existence on Mother Earth. So, we have the sun which feeds and nourishes our life-force; we have the earth on which we are grounded; we have the holy water which flows from our God-head through the chakras of our earthly systems into our ocean of life, and we have the Breath of God. To this recipe of matter we ignite our spirit with the fire, the media through which we live with God. It is through this fire that man must remember his Eternal God, and worship only the All Magnificent, Omniscient Lord God.

"These are the elements of our existence, but how did we evolve? We can turn to the Book of Genesis in the Holy Bible, which narrates the story of man's creation. Adam was the first man and Eve was created from his left rib. The temptations put before Adam by the first woman have been misinterpreted by the evolution of the scriptures. She was the duality of Adam and from the first man and woman the existence of mankind was propagated. The children of Adam and Eve went out into the world and spread the first seed of man through the Grace of God and the blessing of the Divine Father and Divine Mother. The seed was planted in the Garden of Eden and mankind grew into a wide variety of human beings here on earth. This was man's second birth, after the birth of the spark of life caused by God's Finger and the igniting of the sun. This birth gave mankind the Spirit of Life which would then take a second birth through Mother Earth and the Divine Father.

"Adam was a prophet, here to bring the message of the One Eternal God to his children. This message was to be spread throughout the clans of the world, but the story of

Adam and Eve gave way to the density of man's limited capability of thinking. Man soon forgot the promise he made to his Creator to worship only the One Living God. He forgot to look inside for the answers, the right and wrong of the choices of how to live. He succumbed to the temptations of the devil in the material way of things. The laws of man began to prevail to uphold the devil's work, but it was so subtle that man did not recognise the error of his ways. He thought the way to go was by the creation of bigger and better structures of man's own thinking, not the law of nature. He put himself above the wondrous gifts of nature and began to take the life-force out of the natural flow of matter, thus causing imbalance here on Mother Earth. She was the Divine Mother and was abused. She needed the help of the prophets, rasools and angels in order to rectify the damage being done." Babaji pressed on.

"Noah was called by God to build an ark, for there were to be the cleansing floods which would reconstruct the face of the earth. Noah put in his ark all of God's creation, animals of all species in the duality of male and female. Those species which would survive in accordance with the Law of God, Mother Nature and the universe, would be saved through the propagation of Noah's sons, Ham and Sem. Ham was of the sun (hemitic) and Sem was of the moon (semitic). There was a third son of Noah called Japhet, who was the father of the Gogs and Magogs, who are the yellow races and native Americans, including the people of the North Pole. The Tubals were from Japhet and are the Africans. The eating habits of the children of Japhet were not controlled and they ate the flesh of the snake and other animals not in the natural flow of Mother Nature. This caused them to fall to the depths of the devil, once more addicts of worldly living, following their own base instincts rather than that of One-God worshipping. They are the ones to whom mankind is presently bowing, with their weapons of mass destruction and rule of the sword.

"So, there are the children of fire, Ham; the children of water, Sem, and the children of Japhet, the Gogs and Magogs. When the floods abated, the clans of Noah's children dispersed to the mountains and the plains throughout the world, and once more the genesis of man would endeavour to live in the right flow of God's Breath."

Babaji let his words fall into place, before continuing with Abraham's place in the Story of Mankind.

"Abraham was a descendent of Noah through Sem, and was named the father of all mankind, the 12 nations and the father of kings. He was originally named Abram until the day God spoke to him on Mount Thor. God appeared in the guise of a burning fire, the Angel of Fire, and said to Abram:

**Genesis, Chp.XVII, verses 4-7*

4. I Am, and My Covenant is with thee, and thou shalt be a father of many nations.

5. Neither shall thy name be called anymore Abram: but thou shalt be called Abraham: because I have made thee a father of nations.

6. And I will make thee increase exceedingly, and I will make nations of thee, and kings shall come out of thee.

7. And I will establish My Covenant between Me and thee, and between thy seed after thee in their generations, by a perpetual Covenant: to be a God to thee, and to thy seed after thee.

**Taken from Babaji's family Bible which is approximately 200 years. The words differ from that of the modern Bible.*

"Abraham was known as Rama when he lived in India. Ra means the sun and Ma means the moon. Here we have both elements of fire and water evolved from the seed of

Abraham, father of the 12 nations, now known as the 12 signs of the zodiac. Through the seed of Abraham's offspring there are nations of hemitic origin, the sun, and nations of semitic origin, the moon.

"Abraham's first son was Ishmael, whose mother was Hagar. Ishmael was the sentient fountain, which sprang forth from his heel on Mount Thor. This spring is now known as the well at the place of Mecca, a pilgrimage for Moslems. It is also the place where the burning bush appeared to Moses, the Angel of Fire, Lord Raphael, in order to give him the Lord God's Ten Commandments. So, here we have the two elements of water and fire on Mount Thor, where God's Word is perpetuated through the Covenant with Abraham.

"Abraham's second son was Isaac, of semitic descent, born by Sara. Isaac was the Father of Jacob and the grandfather of Joseph, who declared to his elder step-brothers that he was of the sentient fountain, the fountain which spouted from the heel of Ishmael on Mount Thor. Can you see how the family of mankind is growing? It is your heritage. When Joseph was sold as a slave to the Egyptian Queen, Nefertiti, the likeness of Hagar was seen in his face and so he was made Pharaoh of Egypt. The likeness is that of Babaji, as you will see from the photograph of me with the hair flowing behind my back, like the headgear of the Sphinx.

"The heritage of man is to be recognised within you. Please see within, which branch you are from, as it is important that you see the path of your God-given map or blueprint. It will reveal the secrets of your past lessons and guide your future footsteps along the highway to God. These lessons are the way forward and offer spiritual growth to each individual, easing the flow for all members of the family tree. When you look at your own past lives, it affects the lessons of others. The soul essence of your family clan will be cleansed through you. The spirit of your lineage is recovered towards God."

Babaji wanted to aim one more arrow into the hearts of his attending devotees, who were amazed at the unfolding of this ancient story.

"Who are you? You are the beloved image of God and are eternal beings. The Way of God is simple. The complexity of man's ways interferes with the process of self-realisation, and self-realisation leads to God-realisation. Man's ways need to be washed away so that the art of existence can be integrated into everyday living. Obey the Law God, the Ten Commandments, and you will not fail."

Introspection: The Pranayama

The people of Babaji had been sitting in the shade of the larch trees for an hour now. The green energy of these beings infiltrated the ambience of the blessings given by the angels, and all was well. When the full charge of blessings had reached the inner hearts of each and every person, then Babaji would continue his words of wisdom. His disciples were the instruments of his mission and he would not fail in giving them all that they needed to realise themselves. These were the End of Days and he was the orchestrator of the chosen beings in order that man's seed could be saved. Their work was to deliver his lessons to the populations of the world, to garden the weeds out and strengthen the bloodline of mankind. No more would the greed and selfishness of man's unrepentant actions be allowed to ravage the eco system of Mother Earth. She was to be flattened and the sun would diminish. The strong seed of God's creation would be salvaged and the rest would perish. It was the Law of God, which could not be diverted. It was the Law of Cause and Effect.

Babaji watched the individuals. Some were attentive and some were there just for his healing aura. There was a mixture of requirements this day and he would ensure each person received their daily bread.

"How do you know which bloodline is yours? Which way do you search? There are many ways to do this work, my children, and the quickest way is through the kriyas. The kriya yoga is the most direct way to self-realisation. Go deep within, into the core of your being. Be still, be calm, and do nothing. God will pass the veils of forgetfulness which drift in and out of each person's passage of life. He will whisper in your ear the story of your bloodline."

One eagre student interjected at this point, "But how do we know when it is God's voice that we hear and not a voice of our making?" It was clear to Babaji that his words needed more illustration and he showed the correct method of breathing to his class.

Pranayama – Tantra 564 from the book of "Thirumandiram, A Classic of Yoga and Tantra Vol. 1." By Siddhar Thirumoolar.

Master the Steed of Breath

The mind is, the master of senses five;
He is the head of the body habitat;
There is a steed he rides to his destined goal;
The masterly one the steed carries,
The feeble one it throws away;
That steed the Prana breath is.

His class practised the art of this pranayama breath, bringing the breath up to the soft centre of the throat below the adam's apple, locking it into position, then pushing the energy into the head, the pineal, and holding the breath momentarily before pushing the breath back down on the out-breath. The process takes the prana energy up the back along the spine and then down the front of the body, back to the mooladhara, the base chakra. Soon the class was breathing the Breath of Life as it should be, as God intended, as the Food of God. The prana was a life-force on which the body replenishes its daily energies just as much as the living food of the green energy.

"When this kriya is practised and accomplished," Babaji continued, "then naturally we go into meditation, when all is illuminated from our consciousness and God's Voice rings sweetly in our ears. He will reveal the path of life and its course of time to each individual. He will reveal the line of your blood on which you travelled to this point, on your way back to God. He is the Eternal and Infinite One God Whom you are part of. He made man in His own image. The image of man is the mirror of God. Imagine that! We are of God and we struggle and strain to remember the path of our own blood. Let there be no more striving. Breath in the prana and remember your heritage. The Grace of God is upon you. REMEMBER."

The air became still and the angels once more did their work at the instruction of Babaji. Each member of his class would be blessed.

Baptism of Fire

Babaji contemplated the struggle of man's own making, purely because he was intent on making his own path rather than follow the Righteous Path, the Law of God. He saw how each person was affected by the actions of others, how each individual lived accordingly, in order to avoid facing his own music. It seemed to be the line of least resistance for those who were carried along the tide of man's worldly life. There were those who chose to rule with the sword, be it in battle or in the justice courts, and there were those who followed without question. They were the wolves and the sheep. Once more, Babaji would reiterate the way of right living, without the need of another's interpretations. He would show, once more, the art of living by one's own consciousness, in the flow of nature and in step with the Law of God.

He rose from his bed and prepared himself for his day's work. The sun shone brightly and the clouds reflected the essence of this day. The angels were gathering, too, to ensure that they took full opportunity of performing their Creator's instruction, to aid and support each and every man, woman and child in their trials and tribulations of life. There were so many angels that all present at the ashram would be sustained in the lifestyle of God's choosing, not man's own. The people were Babaji's chosen beings and needed all help of Mother Earth, the trees, plants and herbs, the green living energy.

The crowd gathered around the fire pit. There was to be a fire sacrifice that day. The planets were in alignment and the moon and sun at their highest potency for such sacrifice to be performed. This was a day for rejoicement. The fire would ignite the doors in each person so that initiation could be given by Babaji. All would be touched by the living flame's sun energy as they responded in the ritual of vedic chanting. As the sun got into position the ceremony began. Everyone was given some samidha, fire food for the angels, to throw into the flames as the chanting continued in ever increasing momentum. The rhythm of

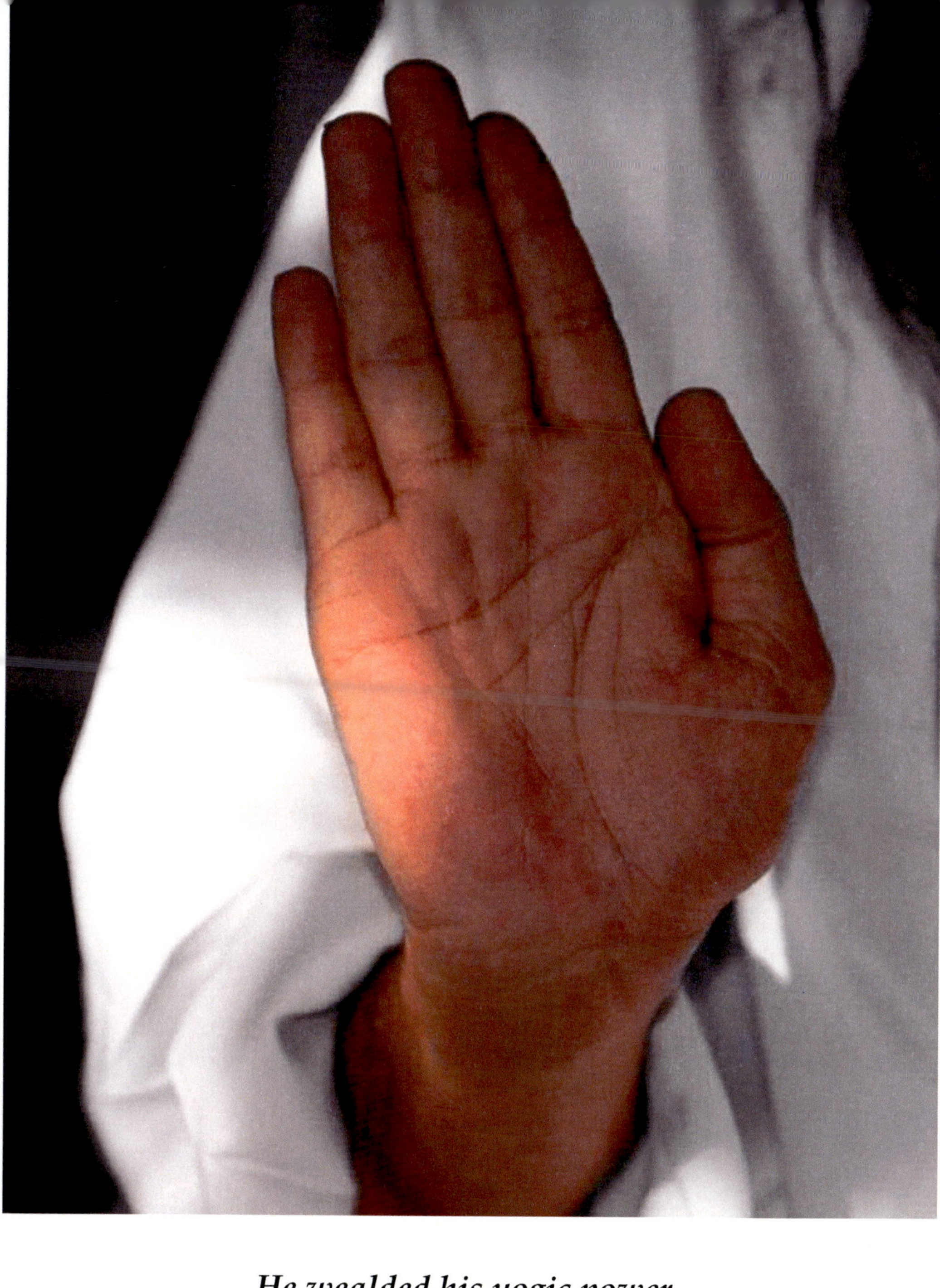

He wealded his yogic power.

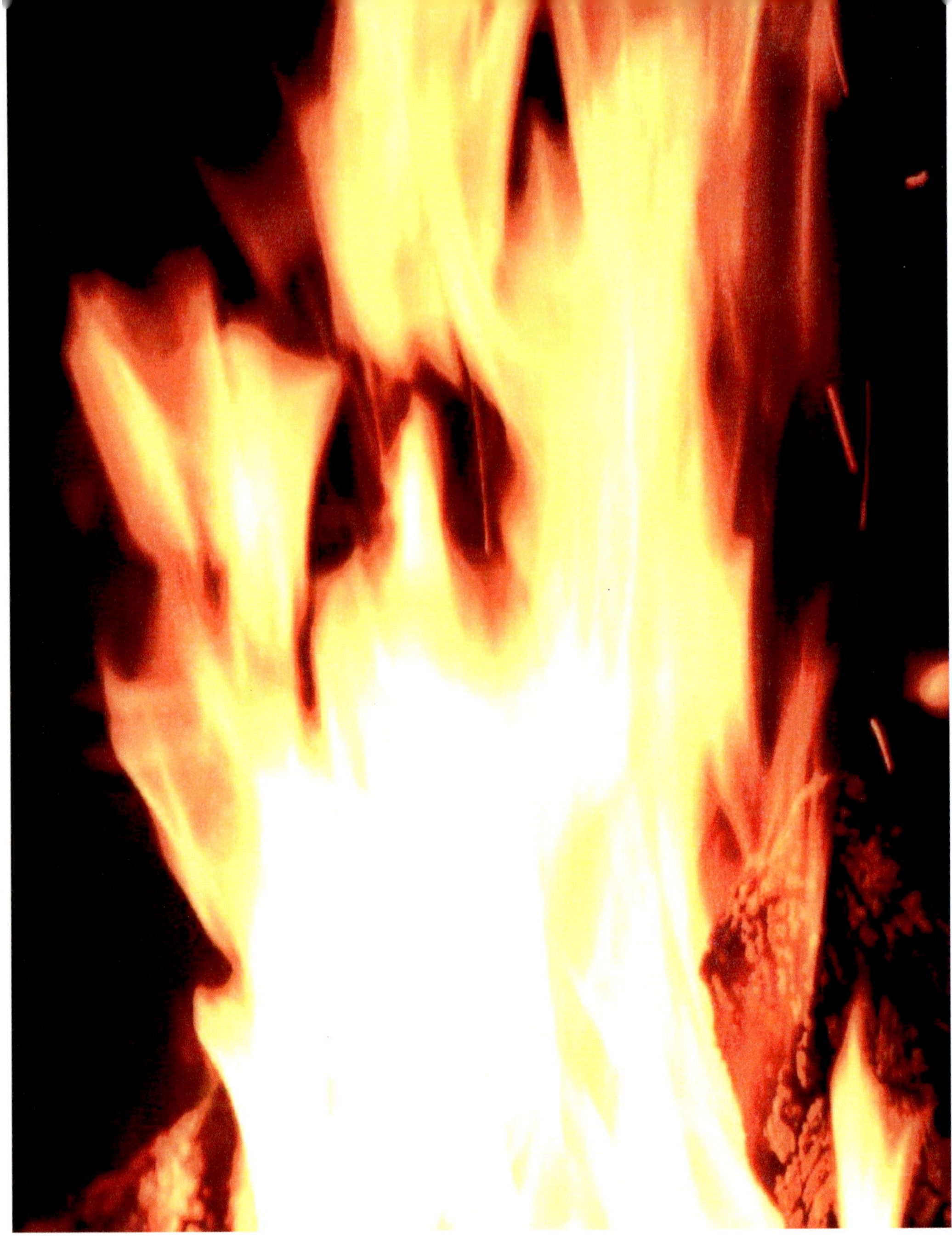

The Angels of fire were in the air.

the words wove its magic as the flames licked ever higher, forming images of God's Word which impregnated each soul. This was a very special ritual of Hindu tradition,

and although Babaji did not aspire to this particular faith, he always took the force of the true aspects of any faith and used its loving energies for the highest good of all. The high vibrational frequencies of the fire was to be choreographed with precision if its fullest potential was to be appreciated. The dancing of the fire was in the powerful hands of a master. Babaji used the tools of his mission with great care and without compunction. He wealded his yogic power only for the higher good, never for anything less than God's work.

Everyone's face glowed with the heat of the fire, which was being replenished with more wood so that its flames once more reached out to great heights. More samidha was distributed to the gathering to continue the magic of their individual responses. The ritual reached its climax and the energies began to come down slowly, gently. It was important not to stop the procedure abruptly. Then came the time for the disciples to make their own way from the fire to a place of quiet repose. Their crown chakras were fully open and in receptive mode. They would feel the full impact of Babaji's initiation of fire within the next moments or perhaps days. All would be blessed with spiritual growth with the hallmark of Babaji. The angels of fire were in the air and the disciples breathed them in. The angelic energies reached the parts that had not seen daylight in eons. More than likely there would be pain experienced by some, before rejoicement. It all depended on their individual healing processes.

After a while Babaji called his disciples to him. He wanted to impart a little more insight to them just as they were in this state of consciousness. Their sensitive state would make this part of the initiation an elixir of life which was to be relished. They would remember this day with their

Master. Babaji gently rested his eyes upon each person and, as he did so, a sense of peace invaded the individual's whole body, linking him forever with the higher frequencies of the fire angels. The Baptism of Fire was completed in a most powerful of initiations. The system of the fire initiation was that of the sun and its higher notes were to be utilised with great care. Only those who Babaji chose to be messengers of his mission would be tuned in this way, together with the loving energies of those working in the higher realms. They would oversee the burdens carried by the chosen ones, and assist in all things to ease the difficulties taken on with the work of the messengers, the tillers of God's Garden.

"Please read the words of the poet, Kahlil Gibran," Babaji advised. "They will heal all ills and pass on the loving experiences of another who walked before you on the path to God. He was the epitome of how life should be lived, an instrument of the Almighty. The writings of this man give all instruction for daily living, without the dogma of man's religious fanaticism. His work has been brought into being for the benefit of all mankind, Hindu, Jew, Christian, Moslem, the like. Please take the opportunity of the vibration of his words.

Quote from 'The Prophet' by Kahlil Gibran:

"Oftentimes have I heard you speak of one who commits a wrong as though he were not one of you, but a stranger unto you and an intruder upon your world. But I say that even as the holy and righteous cannot rise beyond the highest which is in each of you, so the wicked and the weak cannot fall lower than the lowest which is also in you. And as a single leaf turns not yellow but with the silent knowledge of the whole tree, so the wrong-doer cannot do wrong without the hidden will of you all."

"The time is drawing nigh for you to disperse throughout the world with my message of the importance of One-God worshipping. It is as simple as that, but you will experience resistance. Do no fall down at the first sight of obstruction. Be strong and ask God to guide you in all direction. He will ensure you will not fail in your chosen path. Be the example to those who are not able to see for themselves. Let them follow the footsteps of the chosen ones if they refuse any other message of God's making. They will ride the tide of change by the pull of your light. Shine your beacon from the very end of the land and mountain tops. I am the cry on the mountain. Echo my cry and the magnet will pull in with the magnificent forces of the Eternal God, the Creator of ALL."

The faces of his disciples reflected the enormity of what was being entrusted to them. Put in the staged words of Babaji it seemed a task of such magnitude. The infrastructure of God's work was sound. The gifted beings would do his work unerringly.

The Ten Commandments

Moses came to Mount Thor and the burning bush spoke to him, the Angel of Fire. He spoke God's Word to him and gave him the Ten Commandments. Moses was entrusted with leading his people back into the lap of God's Law, the way of cause and effect. They are the commandments by which mankind has endeavoured to abide by. There are those who succeed, but it is the mission of Babaji, as it was the mission of Moses, to gather back the ones who have strayed through following the laws of man's own making, the laws which have been bent to suit the greed and need of worldly living.

Babaji wanted to clarify the Ten Commandments to his people, to show them how God's Law was tantamount to walking in the natural flow of nature. He decided to use the energies of the fuchsia growing in and around his ashram grounds. The properties of this particular flower were that of cellular regrowth. All past sins of man could be repayed by future generations in order to rebalance the karmic balance sheet within him. The structure of the flower was to release the seeds of doubt in the most beneficial manner of each individual and could be done through the dance of life, the path of the individual. The colours of the different varieties of fuchsia in the ashram's gardens would also enable all shades of light in the hues of mauve and magenta to seep through the grades of density of sin. This grace of Mother Nature, the Divine Mother, had the strength to rectify the balance of wrong and right doing. It would aid in the transformation from worldly living to that of the natural flow with the positive cosmic energy in the whole of creation.

The rug had been placed at the foot of the steps where Babaji liked to sit before his people, in the full energy of the sun. There were seats, too, along the front of the ashram, and the fuchsias hung in elegant singularity from the bushes spread along the frontage. The people wandered into the grounds quietly, drinking in the energies of Babaji as soon as they stepped through the ashram gates.

The flowing colours of the saris and gowns of the ladies gave a weave of energy, creating the unique consistency of the day's work for Babaji. He felt the requirements of his people build before him in the meld of the day's words. Some would need the power of definite instruction and others would gently adjust their daily lifestyle according to their own consciousness. Everyone lived by their own consciousness, but some were not so awake in their inner wisdom. These were the people who would be spood-fed the Ten Commandments.

He pointed out the fuchsias glowing around the garden and gave thanks to the Lord God for their singular beauty. The Lord God was showing the people how to BE within the full picture of a living situation, and the flowers were equal among them. They shone out their healing rays and all were in receipt of God's Blessing. These blessings happened all the time, and the art of living was to appreciate God's Food when it was placed before an individual, a group of people or the immense population of a civilisation.

Babaji loved his plants and regularly walked through his garden of herbs, plucking the leaves of particular plants, saying to whoever was close by, "Eat it! It will be good for you. The quality of this plant will revive the energy within you if you wish to help your systems adjust to a more healthy state. It's rather like servicing your motor car which has been running on the same dirty, used oil for the past 6 months. It is good to use the free things in life for this purpose. It is the Breath of Life."

Babaji's words began to flow. His theme would be the story of Moses, how he came into this world and was placed in a situation of responsibility for the children of Israel, how he guided them away from the deadly masters of the sword, the wolves.

**Exodus, Chp III, verses 14 & 15*

14. God said to Moses: I Am Who Am. He said: Thus shalt thou say to the children of Israel: He Who Is, hath sent me to you.

15. And God said again to Moses: Thus shalt you say to the children of Israel: The Lord God of your fathers, the God of Abraham, the God of Isaac, and the God of Jacob hath sent me to you: this is My Name for ever, and this is My Memorial unto all generations.

**Taken from Babaji's 200 year old family Bible.*

"So, Moses did as God had directed and led his people into the wilderness where they spoke of their doubts of their leader's wisdom in bringing them there. At least they were fed and watered by their old masters of the sword, they said to him. Moses was a prophet, sent once more to bring the seed of man back into the natural flow of things. He was to be given the Word of God in order to give the people the written guide-lines of a righteous living, the path home to the One Omniscient Living God.

"When the people said to Moses that they no longer wanted to follow him, he left them and made his own way to the place where he knew his ancestors had received the revelations of God. He went to Mount Thor, the same as Abraham, the father of nations and kings, where he, himself, was to be given the Ten Commandments by the Lord of Fire, Raphael. God said only one word to Moses, 'Jahweh', 'I Am'. The vibration of this one word is the whole thing, but the commandments have been misinterpreted and given meaning according to mankind's own consciousness, but I will set out for you the true meaning of the Laws of God as they were intended to be used.

"Firstly, you worship the One God. Do not worship the

puppets and idols of man's own making. Do not worship the prophets who have come to give you the path. They are there to guide you towards the Eternal God, to be the eternal beings that you are. Worship only Him Who Is, the Immortal and Invisible Lord God. Live for the Eternity of God, not the doomed destiny of man's worldly living. Man is not God. God Is God. Man is here for a short tenure only on this smallest of living planets, which has been given by the Creator for man's spiritual growth. Give praise to the One Who gives life, not the lords and gods of unsustainable living. He is the One to Whom we should turn in our hour of need, and He will be merciful to those who hold the Lord God in the rightful place in their hearts and souls. Whether you are Moslem, Jew, Christian or Hindu, worship the One God of all creation, not the dead relics of the religions. Carry forward the love of the prophets, but only adore the Almighty, Himself. Do not misuse the Name of God. He is the Creator of all things and is the Truth. This is the essence of life itself. Do this and you will not fail in walking the path home to God."

Babaji paused to emphasize the power of his words, and then continued to reiterate the importance of One-God worshipping.

"Keep a day holy for the Sabbath. If you are a Moslem it is Friday; if you are a Jew it is Saturday and if you are a Christian it is Sunday. Keep yourself clean inside and out and dedicate this day to the worshipping of God Almighty. Leave your tasks and worldly things aside and concentrate your thoughts and prayers towards the Everlasting God, He Who loves you. Be careful what you eat in honour of the Lord God. Eat no meat or fish, but eat the fruits and harvest of Mother Nature. Nor must you eat any reproductive yeast, but keep yourself wholesome and clean.

"Next: Honour thy mother and father. Pay respect to them. They are your worldly guides and, as such, will serve you with all lessons of growing up from an infant into childhood, when you start to develop your own level of knowingness. Even though you may differ in your vibrational thinking when you grow in your own wisdom, still you should pay the respect to your earthly parents. Love and cherish them always. They have done their very best to nurture you in the best possible way."

The next commandment needed absolute clarification for the good of his mission, 'Nor kill'.

"This commandment is quite clear, 'Nor kill'. Man has interpreted this as, 'Do not kill if it is not necessary.' God was quite categorical about killing. It means do not kill any living being, even if it is a small insect or small animal. Give life to others and you shall be given life. Of course, there are times when an insect is killed unknowingly, and this sin is forgiven when cleansing before and after prayer. This sin is taken away by the Lord God and written off the balance sheet before your Day of Reckoning. But the Lord God did not intend that man eat the flesh of animals, thereby living at the same level of consciousness as the animals, themselves. You are not dogs in the street, but a human being with the inner wisdom. When you search inside for your own answers about God, you will realise that the Food of God is not the flesh or the fish, but the God-given energy of plants, the green energy. Be a good vegetarian and do not drink the intoxicating liquour which addles the brain. This is not a clean way of living. The same accounts for drugs which also make you mad. Live a clean life within the structure of Mother Earth's bounteous store of light food, within the flow of the Law of God.

"Do not commit adultery. This is a big sin. It means do not go to any man or woman who is married or promised to be married. If you are married or betrothed, do not go to another man or woman. Be faithful to your husband or wife. If you go to a woman or man and promise to marry them, then this is permissible. Make your oath to join

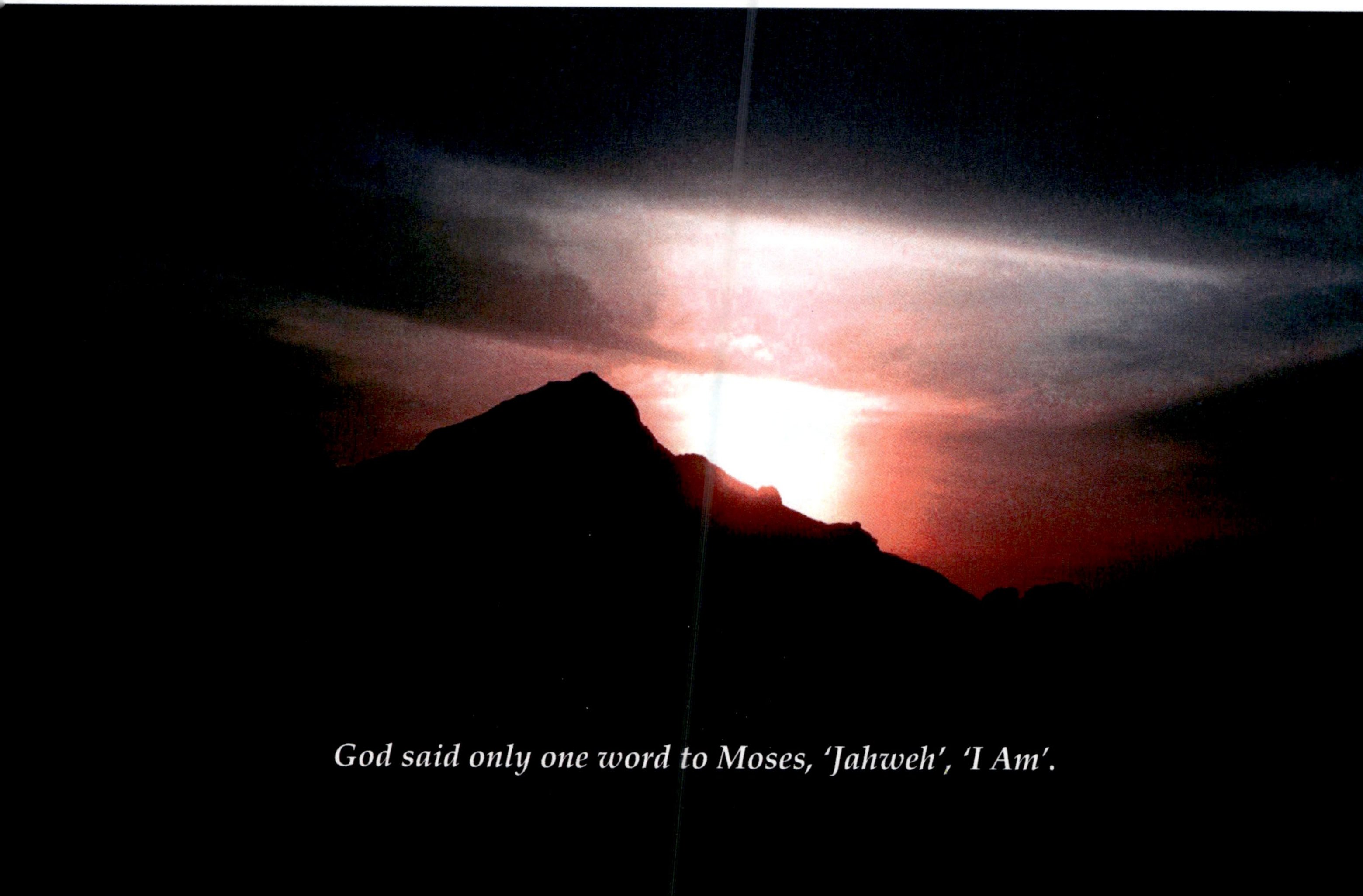

God said only one word to Moses, 'Jahweh', 'I Am'.

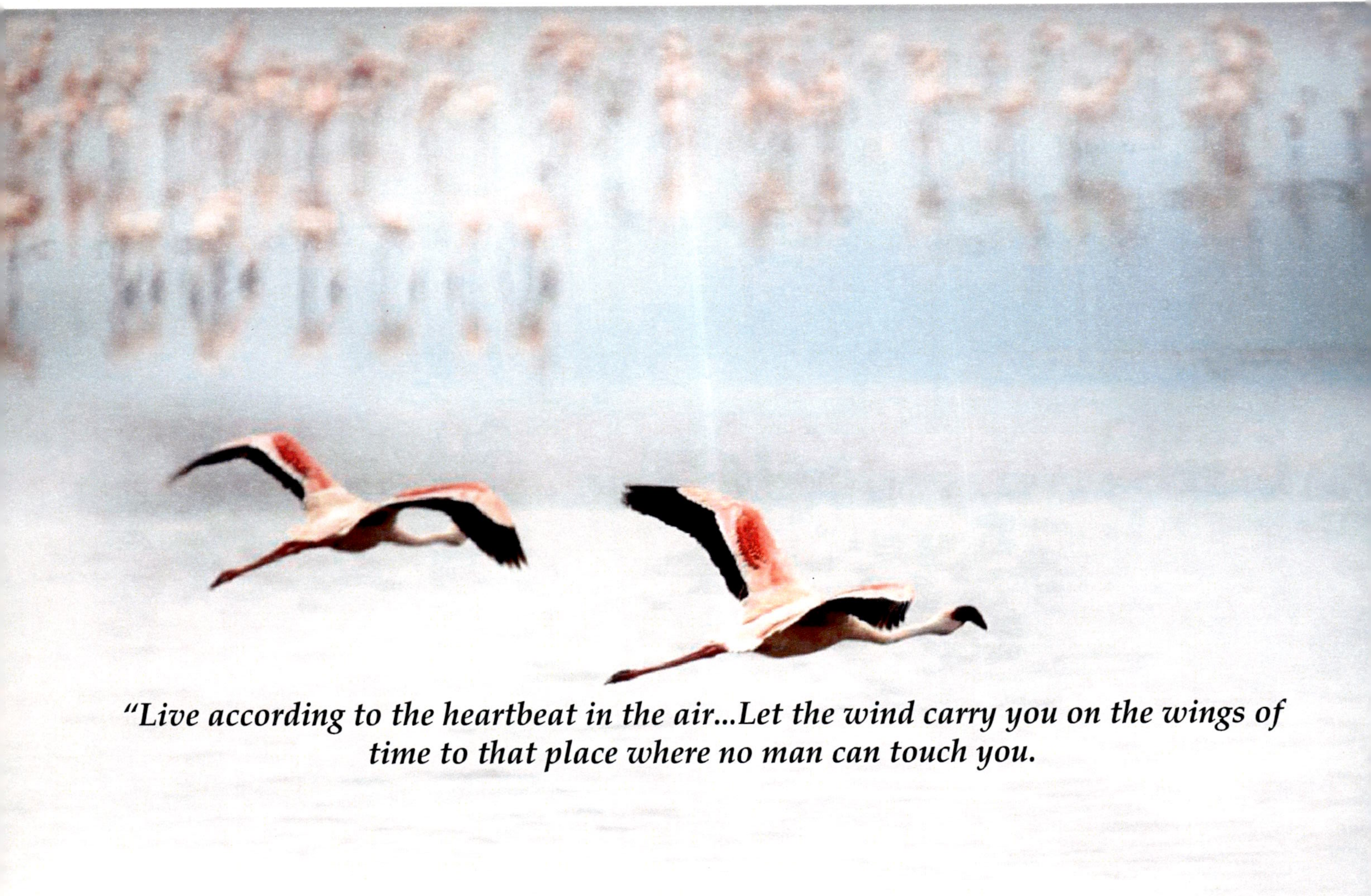
"Live according to the heartbeat in the air...Let the wind carry you on the wings of
time to that place where no man can touch you.

together as man and wife before God, but if you wish to go to another partner, then divorce is necessary. However, it is better to be faithful to one person in the Eyes of God.

"If you go to your brother, mother, father or sister, this is a most unforgivable sin, because it is anti-nature. The seed of man must be protected and this sin is in direct contra-flow to the continuation of man's existence. God's Garden must be kept weeded at all times so that its harvest will thrive. Living in such sin will cause the seed of man to deviate towards the devil. The debts of the ancestors will be a heavy burden on the shoulders of the offspring of such issue.

"Next: Love thy neighbour and live in community. It was the custom of Abraham to offer hospitality to strangers who visited his neighbourhood. He would ensure that they were given food and drink by his family, and offered the hand of friendship to all. So, follow the tradition of your forefathers. Do unto others as you would have done unto you. If you have food only sufficient for yourself, give it to the hungry person in the street, give him warmth. If you do good towards others, you shall receive back goodness and mercy.

"Do not covet the things of others. Have the charity within you and you will be rewarded. It is the Law of God.

"Do not steal from your neighbour, nor charge interest on any loan you may make. Let the natural flow of the money energy take its own course and you will be recompensed in the right order of things. It is the law of the universe, God's Law of Cause and Effect.

"Do not interfere with your neighbour's life-force. This means do not tell untruths about him, for surely the lies will return to their source and will be accountable in your Book of Life. The truth always makes its presence known.

"You have been born by the Will of God, not by your own will. One day you will return to your Creator and be accountable for your deeds. So, do good, think good, be good and eat good. That, my children, is the art of living."

His people knew that Babaji was their Master and mentor, their Guru, and as such they would follow his example. He only spoke the Word of God, but they could see that there would be hurdles to overcome if they were to adapt to this natural way of living. They would have to face their fears, because not all members of the community would see the light ahead and friction would ensue.

"Babaji, it would be all too easy for us to live in this way if society were as one in its thinking. How do we live by God's Law if the rest of the population is busily abiding by the law of the land, those laws which are imposed upon us by our leaders and politicians?" said one man from the crowd.

"If you bring the Law of God into your own everyday life it will filter into the lives of others. Live by your own consciousness and others will react to the positive nature of your actions. It is the way of things." Babaji continued, "Live according to the heartbeat in the air, like the birds in this tree above you. Let the wind carry you on the wings of time to that place where no man can touch you. The place is within the centre of your being where there is nothing but peace and understanding. With this essence throbbing within you, you cannot be influenced by the wrong-doings of others. Your faith in the Eternal Living God will bring you to the wide open space of good living. The fields and meadows of God's land is available to all. The world at large is there for all. It is God's land, made as the playing fields for all of mankind, and the White Brotherhood is its keeper. If you do good to others, the goodness will be yours. Give resource to this energy and it will increase in its favours. You are the beneficiaries of God's creative stores. Use them when you need them and the cup will be replenished."

Your Friends and Foes

"Your friend is your foe who is teaching you the way," said Babaji. "Never doubt that God will provide the answer in the right order of things. Therefore, before you denounce someone who is not resonating with your own frequency, know that the table of adversity is before you. That is, your strength lies in the way you handle any given situation with ease and comfort.

"When you walk through the valley of the shadow of death, know that the Lord God is by your side, stalking your fears and worries. He will vanquish them from the chambers of your mansion. He will place you in the pastures of green where the still waters are. Here, He will restore your soul without fail. All you must do is follow the Righteous Path in the way given to the prophet, Moses, on God's own mountain, Mount Thor. Remember, the simpler you live, the cleaner the heart. Leave all things of complexity in the refuse bin at the bottom of the mountain. The bin will absorb all things of darkness and be given to the universe as matter for recording by the angels of mercy and compassion. Once recorded, your sins and fears are absolved forever and ever, never to return. This is the Covenant of God."

The air was calm as the Master's words of wisdom sank into the hearts and minds of those around him. There were more questions, he knew, and he waited.

"But what if the people we are living with, and making the rules for our daily lives, are the very people you tell us to honour? What if those people of people's confines are our parents? How do we obey them and still live by our own consciousness?"

"Thy love of your parents is always there, whether you follow their commands or whether you take careful steps to honour your own godhead," responded Babaji. "Live in full accord of the household, but surrender your problems over to God. Pray for the difficulties of loved

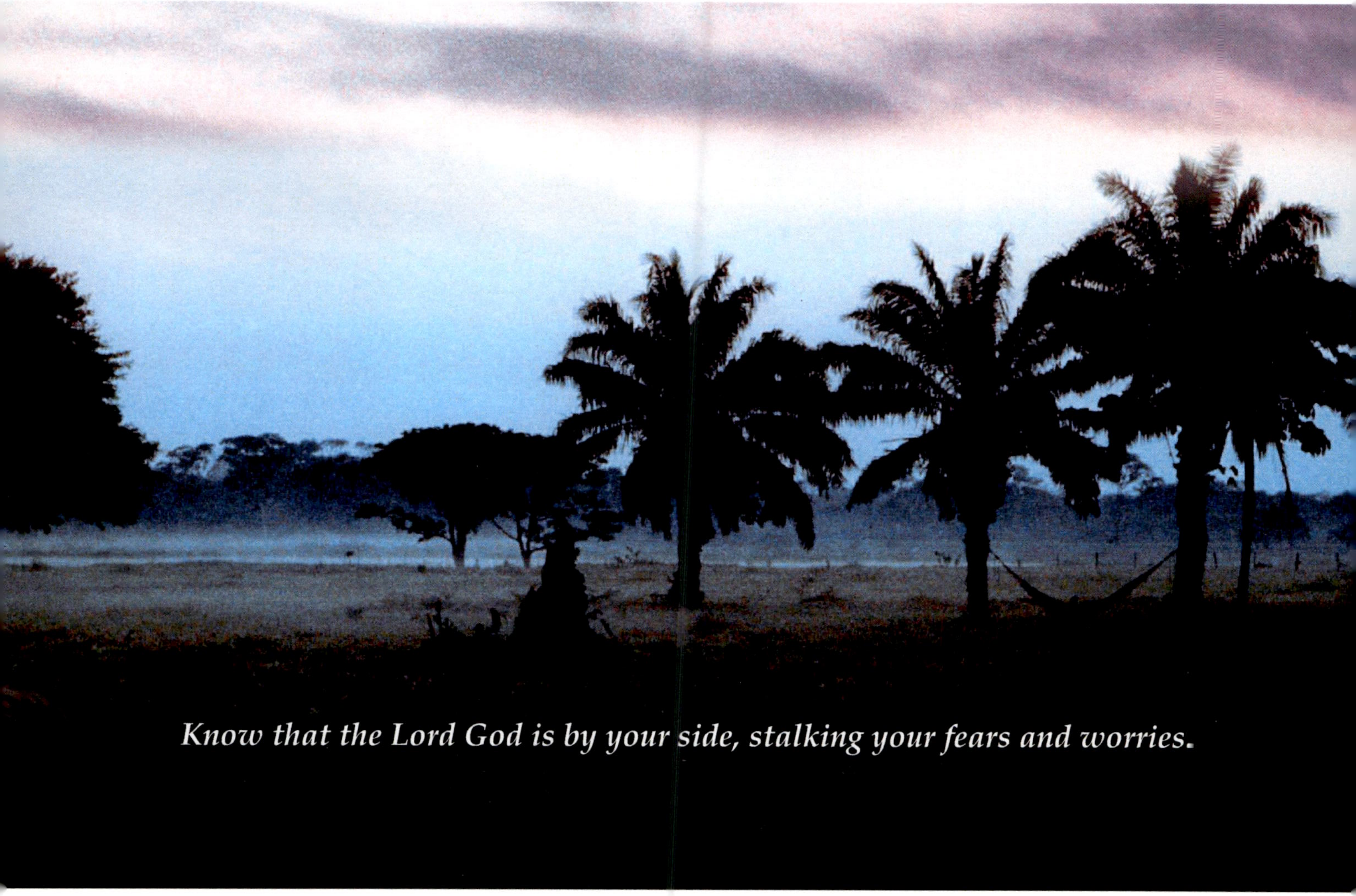
Know that the Lord God is by your side, stalking your fears and worries.

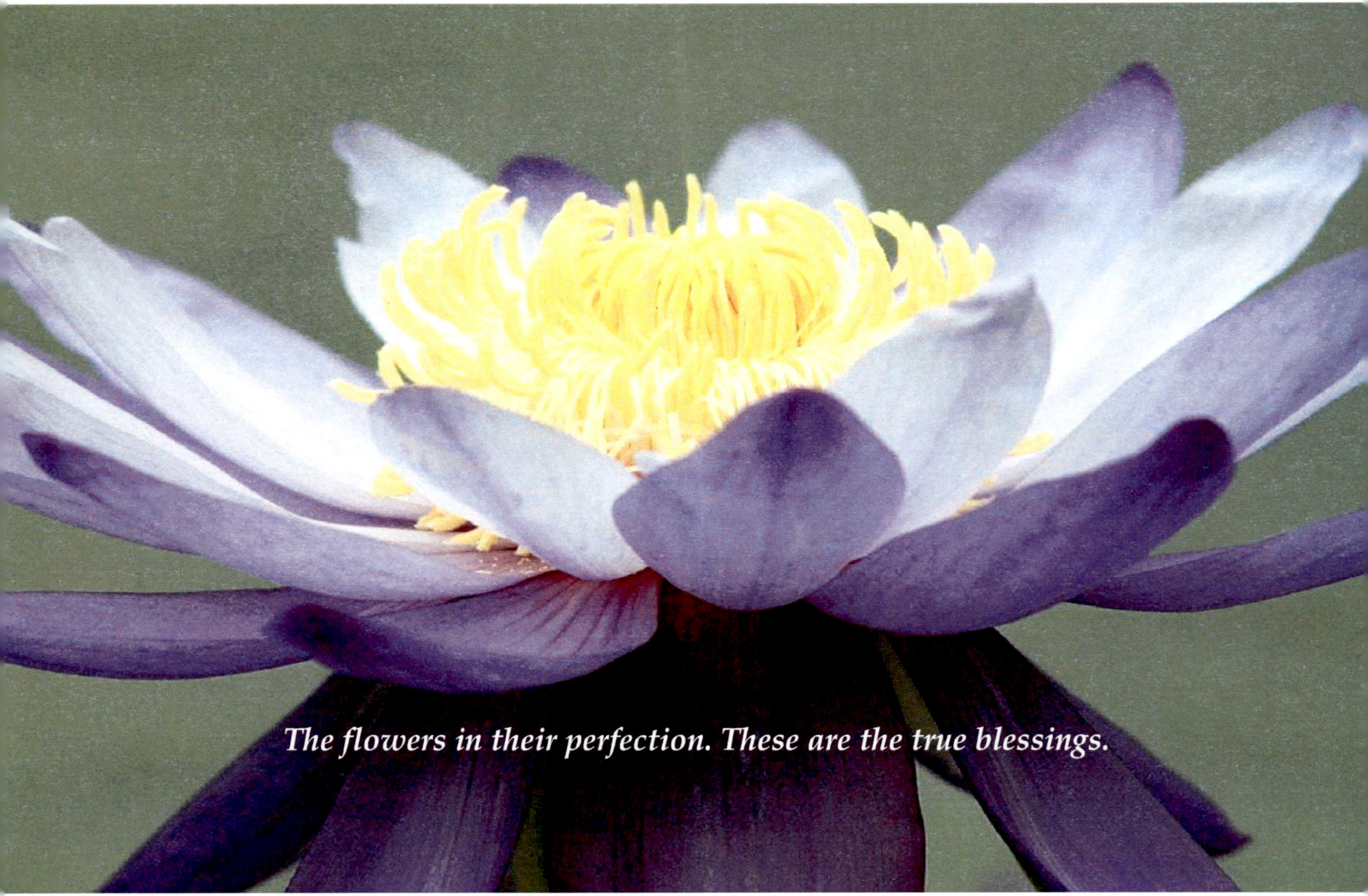
The flowers in their perfection. These are the true blessings.

ones to be overcome. Allow the answers to be given without condition and all will be resolved with the ease and comfort of the All Compassionate One Living God."

"Thank you, Babaji," said the devotee with gratitude. "We will remember to pray for all our friends and family." Then, yet another of life's dilemmas was put to the Guru.

"And what must we do when the truth is not being prevailed, Babaji? Sometimes the words of others are not truthful. Do we live with the energies of such false witness, or do we fight for the truth?"

"Ah, my child, this is a most useful lesson. Learn to let the wrong words or actions of others go. They will soon dissipate into the positive ethers of God. He will tend to the outcome of wrong doings. It is all in the divine running of things, and justice prevails. So, therefore, learn not to be affected by such words and deeds. If you come out of animation, then you no longer are part of any further karmic action. Let go of such idiocy and be part of the divine flow. It is much more peaceful, I assure you. Pray to the Lord God for the unconditional love to envelop the energies of any harmful words which are intent on reaching their mark in the hearts of others. The love of the Divine Mother is the softest and gentlest. She can alleviate the pain and suffering of such action. Pray, pray, pray with the Name of God and all will be well." Another voice ventured out from the crowd.

"What about the jealousies of our neighbours, Babaji? We all like our things around us, the gemstones on our fingers which adorn our bodies, the things which our loving husbands have given as a mark of their love. These things can easily be stolen because they are coveted by others. How do we deal with this element of our neighbours, or even our own desire to have possessions like those of our friends?"

"Yes, my child," said Babaji with compassion. "This is an

element of mankind which leads on to bigger sin. Beware of coveting thy neighbour's belongings. It is a dangerous state of mind. Leave all worldly desires behind and look to God for the free beauty around you. There are many diamonds in the sky, and flashes of light on the water's surface. There are the dewdrops in the grass and on the cobwebs of spiders. There are the rubies within the dancing living flames of your home fire. The snow and ice gives off the sparkling reflections of winter's light. Give thought to the free store of Mother Nature's abundance, the flowers in their perfection and the perfume of the blossom in the trees. See how the dragonfly flashes its emerald green and peacock blue as it darts about the river bank. These are the true blessings which you should wish for and not the material possessions of others. Let the desires of the lower elements of life go. Live with the higher frequencies of your own godhead and allow the burden of all worldly wishes to flow into the oceans of sorrow, to be cleansed and filtered by the healing waterfalls of your inner wisdom.

"Inner reflection is the way to see beyond the burdens of life. Look inside for your own answers and you will be supported by God's helpers, the angels and messengers who are there simply to watch and guide your every action. If you feel that a burden is weighing heavy, then pass it on to His angels. The burden is theirs as soon as you surrender it to them. The call of the angels is the lightest way of rejoicing the Way of God. They filter the density of living, and aid in the footfall of life's burdens. Give them up to the angels and enjoy the day's gift of time. The life is for being. The way is simple and you are a part of it.

"So, remember to walk the path of simplicity in all things that you do. Go, now, my children. Start your next breath and footstep with this in heart and mind and I will see you the morrow." Babaji blew his blessings to the people as they took their leave. Always, he sent them off with a kiss in the air, the kiss of life.

The Listening Ears, The Inner Eyes

When Babaji saw that the day had brought with it a different hue, a different cadence of light, he knew that the season was changing. He could see that the days ahead would provide new opportunity for him to sit before his devotees in a more relaxed ambience. He enjoyed this time of year when the sun dropped a little in the sky. The light was able to infiltrate one's system and offered a gentler healing vibration to the inhabitants of Nainital. The mountains always gave a magnificent range of light as the clouds rolled along the ridges, across the Lake Naini. Maybe he would test his devotees today.

Babaji set up the meditation elements with his Beloved Lord God.

"Dear God, I ask for the angels to really put their light energies into this day with me, as the people of my following arrive for more words of wisdom from You. You are the Greatest Guide, dear Lord, and I ask that You bless my devotees with the insight to look beyond the normal boundaries of their meditation studies. Let them venture further into the realms of higher vibration, where all is one with You. Let them experience the bliss of absolutely nothing here on earth. So be it. It is done."

Even before the devotees took their places in the meditation room, the Breath of God had reached their solar plexus chakras, placed at the heart of their systems, the place where all energies are expanded and ignited by the act of drawing up the spiritual breath of the Holy Spirit, the Breath of God. This breath was the prana on which man could exist in the beautiful flow of nature, without the stress and strain of the material world and its hunger of lower densities, the food of the devil's temptations. The room was so peaceful and each person was able to sit within his own cave, without undue disturbance of others who were still settling into place. There were pictures of Babaji's family and that of the Messiah. Babaji, too, was illustrated sitting in the lotus position, looking towards his third eye

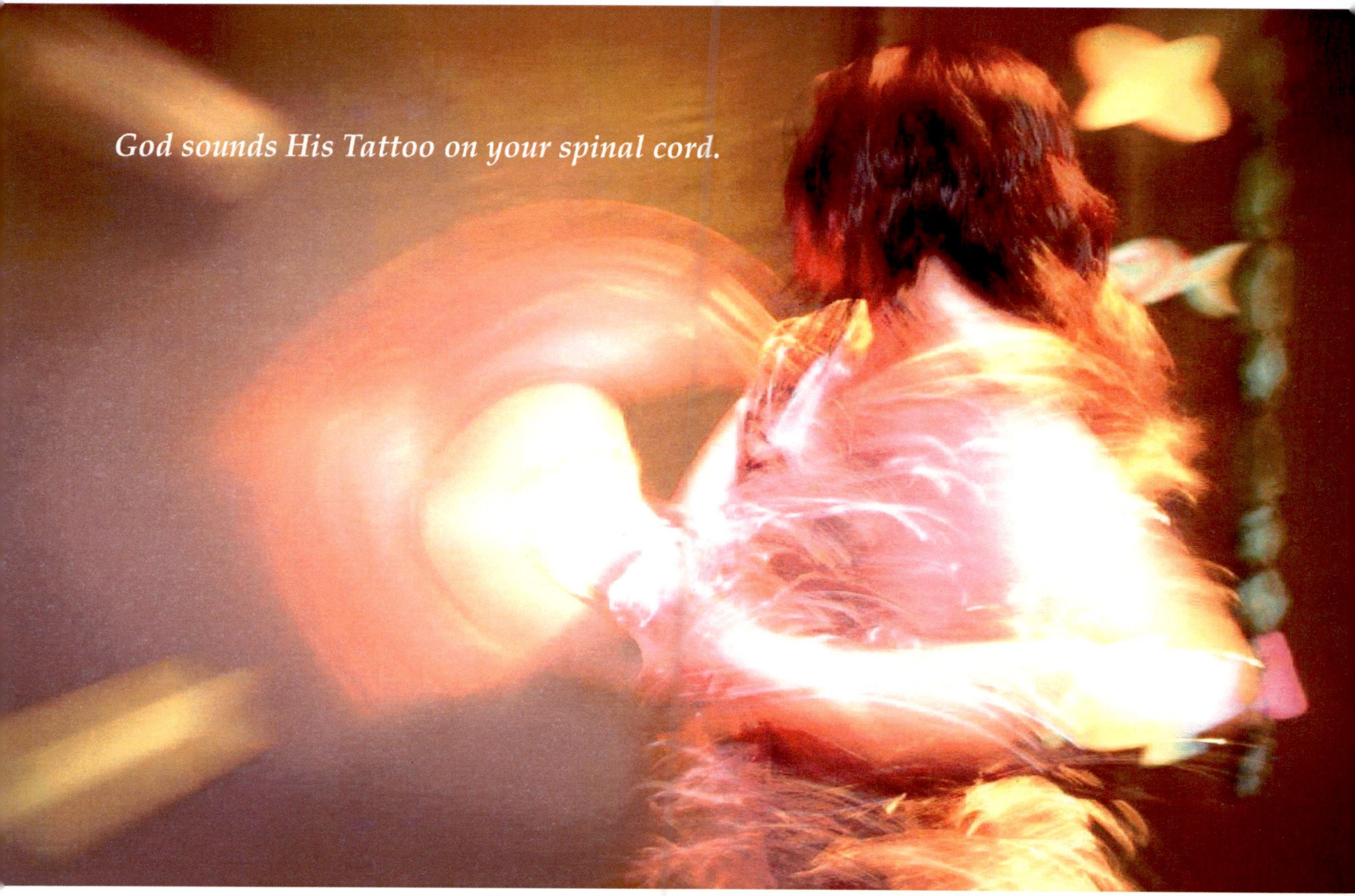
God sounds His Tattoo on your spinal cord.

and seeing his enlightened self. The Divine Mother was ever present and the mix of the heavenly bodies was just divine.

Babaji commenced the lesson and led the class into the kriyas.

"I want you to go within with the aid of the kriyas. Firstly, use the kapalabhati breath to clean the nadis. Then do the bhastrika breath which will stoke up the fire within. The energies of this day can be used for furtherance of your inner wisdom. The sound is in your body and it is possible to listen to the sonographic beating of God's drum. He sounds His Tattoo on your spinal chord, which resonates outwards to all parts of your body: head, feet, shoulders and finger tips. This sonographic sound, or Song of God, is for you to decipher and expand with louder chords of rejoicement. Watch, too, the pattern of life as it emanates from your soul into the universe of infinite wisdom. You can add your own positive energies into the stream of life."

Babaji led the way and demonstrated once more the bhastrika breath, which would take his students into a charged mode. The class fell into his rhythm of breathing and commenced their journey inside. It was interesting to note the variation of breathing of each participant, but Babaji knew their techniques were good. Gradually, the energetic heaving of the bhastrika breath gave way to softer inhalation and exhalation, and the group breathed as one with their Creator. After a time, the sound of God's Song played on the strings of each lute in Babaji's masterful hands. The notes sounded long and drifted further and further into the inner realms. The devotees were able to ride the waves of vibration until they passed the limits of their previous experiences in meditation. The music moved on and on, without the interference of the mind, questioning this or that, wondering what the point of no return was. There was no point of return, but the experiences of each person was to provide him with the potential to let go of all boundaries. The limited thoughts of man was a huge hurdle for him to straddle, but it was within the grasp of everyone in the meditation room that day. One by one, Babaji accorded the appropriate level of understanding to his group. They would each attain the heights of their individual requirements and take huge steps towards God-realisation. If they could listen to their own song, singing in harmony with the rest of creation, then they could reach ever further into the store of inner wisdom, with its infinite depths of God's qualities within them.

"Hold no boundaries within your hearts and you will receive the riches of God-living." Babaji dropped this final pearl of wisdom into his devotee's laps as they began to come round from the higher frequency of introspection, back into the peaceful environment of the meditation room. Another blessing had been bestowed upon them.

Gifts From Babaji

His regular followers fell into place in their blessed routine of visiting the ashram, meditation, prayer and kriya yoga practise. They intermingled with the patients who came for Babaji's medicines and spiritual healing. Some of his disciples had been initiated into performing the healing rituals using the Word of God and the magical healing words of the Suurahs in the Koran. These disciples were much revered by the Indian patients, who often blessed the healer before leaving the ashram.

The people came with a wide spectrum of ails, including the negative influences of the occult, ghosts and malevolent spirits. These would be dealt with by the use of a large bunch of bichhu *(Hindi word)* leaves, very similar to the stinging nettle, but somehow they had a much, much stronger sting and could be very painful to endure. This plant would beat out the ghost together with the use of holy water, peacock feathers and the Suurah Jinn from the Koran. The bichhu leaves also worked in much the same manner as Chinese acupuncture to alleviate the pain from sources of problems such as the inner workings of the life systems of the body, or the damaged joints of old age. The peacock feathers would be swept around the aura of the patient which would clean the outer bodies as the healing within took place. Holy water would be sprinkled over the patient as the Name of God or an appropriate Suurah was recited. Beautiful brass bowls with the God's Name inscribed inside the bowl were filled with water, and the water adopted the vibration of His Name before being used on the patient. It never failed. The Word of God was all powerful.

Such was the regular work at the ashram. The servants cleaned and prepared the ashram for visitors, the cook prepared fresh food on the open fire of the outside cookhouse, the dispensers of the herbal remedies and homeopathic medicines were ready to keep the flow of patients supplied, explaining to them how the medicines should be taken. The western devotees would spend their

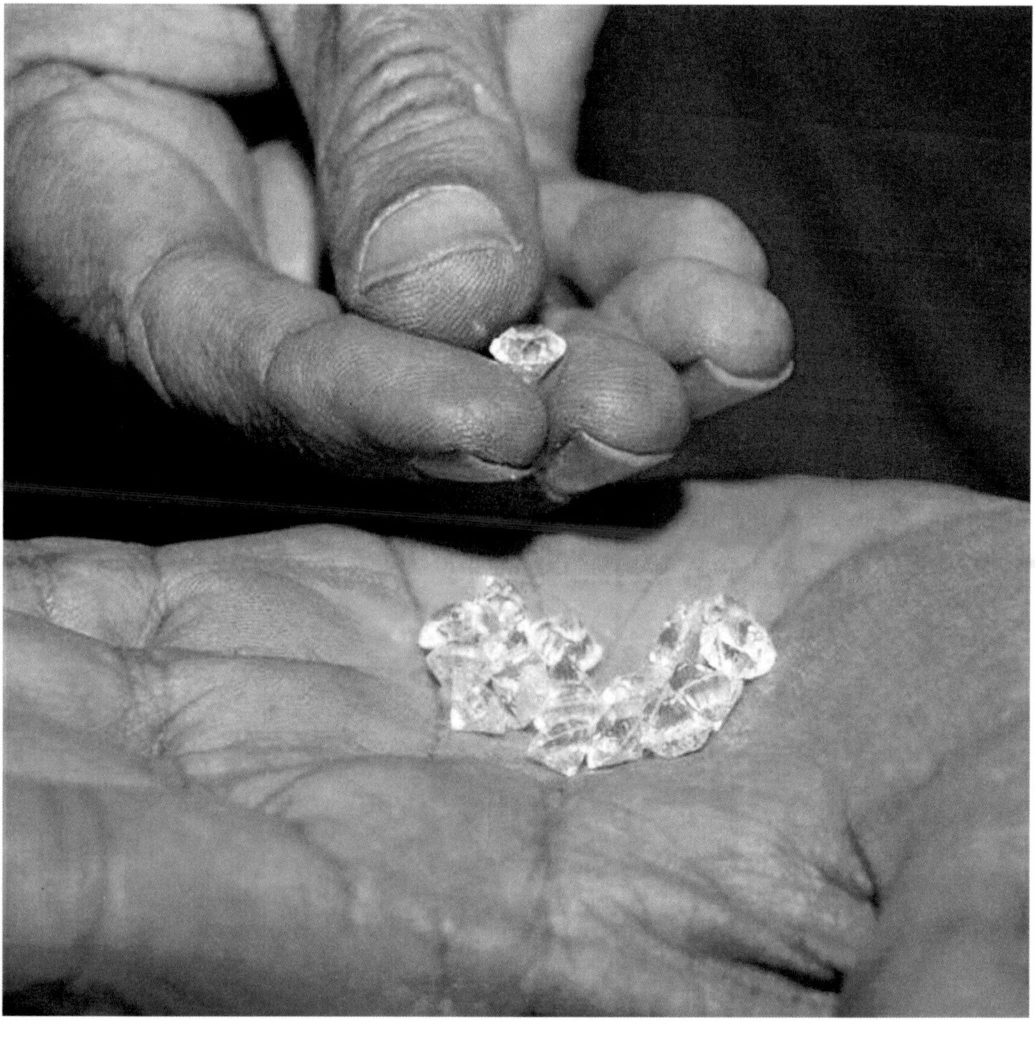

There were gemstones and pendants which they could wear as a constant reminder of who was their Master.

time in meditation, also bringing positive vibrations into the ashram. These were the gifts of Babaji.

At the end of one such day, the patients had dispersed, the late afternoon sun shone on the ashram steps and the small group of disciples sat around their beloved Babaji, just enjoying his wonderful aura around them. They were blessed with the sun energy as well as Babaji's words of wisdom. He never failed to repeat and repeat the importance of thanking the Lord God for each and every blessing of the day and the disciples revelled in his words. The Master took from his room the gifts he wished to pass on to his disciples that day. There were gemstones and pendants which they could wear as a constant reminder of who was their Master. The gems would always reflect the recipient's path and aid the way forward for them. Some received a simple rudraksha seed containing the Name of God written in the formation of the seed. The seed worked on the brain and enabled the wearer to live with the clarity of mind, receiving messages from God and His messengers on how to walk the Righteous Path.

"You are my gardeners," said Babaji, "and will show the path to those scattered around the world. You are my chosen beings, the gifted beings, who will heal the rift between East and West. With me, you will build the bridge of friendship between the religions. You will reflect the way to live in the flow of nature to the rest of the world. You are my seed and that of Ishmael, the sentient fountain. The way is being prepared for the second coming of Christ and you will be positioned to play your part along his side."

The Flaming Torch Within

"The torch within you is given to you by baptism of fire, the initiation of Babaji," Babaji continued. "This blessing is the media used by your Babaji, because it is a frequency related to the burning bush on Mount Thor, where the Archangel Raphael appeared to Hagar, mother of Ishmael. Ishmael was the sentient fountain from where the prophet, Jesus, comes. The water with the fire is the alchemy of life.

"Jesus said, 'I am from my Father in heaven, come to give succour to mankind in his hour of need. The way of man is to wander this way and that, but he is programmed by the Almighty God to *come unto me on the Path of Righteousness.*'

"Man is heading towards disaster, even though he knows the way to go. Fear not, for you shall be kept on the rightful path. The fire and water are the elements which work the frequencies of cleansing. They fill the void created when good work has been done, but they need to be ignited and poured in just the correct manner so that the created energy is flowing freely into the crevices of the mindset of those who do not wish to travel in the best mode. The torch is to be used by masters of fire and water. Be one of the masters and choreograph the path of Jesus.

"Thus spoke the Lord God to the masters. Be guides to those who are blind and deaf to the way of the One Omniscient God. They know not what they do, but influence the road to ruin in just a small movement of their finger. So, harness the power of the elements within, and drive the locomotive engine smoothly. There are many carriages attached to this train and any number of people can climb aboard. The engine must be stoked up at all times in order to maintain the momentum of God's vehicle to eternity. Be responsible for your followers, those who trust in your process without question, those who live intently in accordance with the way of their ancestors, because that is what they have been taught and that is what they know. Be responsible for the gems of life in your

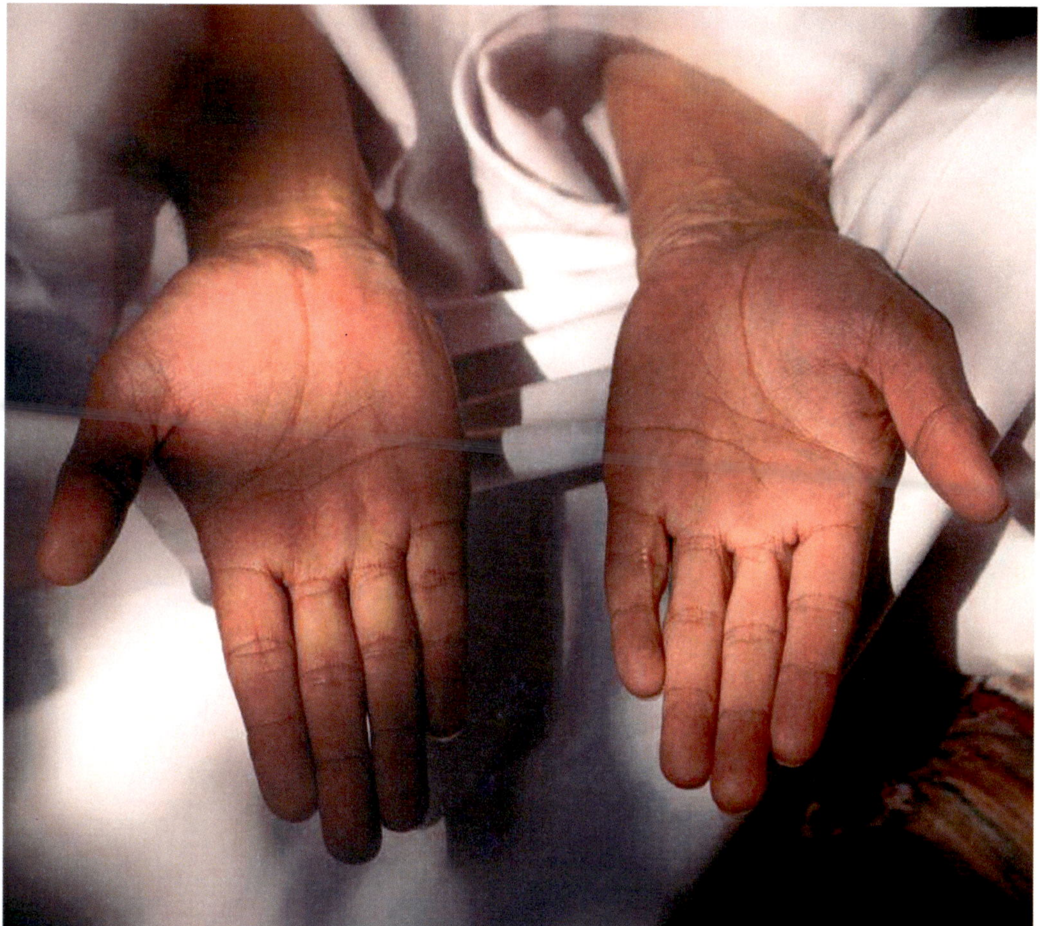

Be responsible for the gems of life in your hands. They will not fail if used for the highest good of all.

ands. They will not fail if used for the highest good of all. The power is so great, but do not fear the work it brings to the drivers of such energy. The rewards are equally great and freedom shall be yours.

"If you prepare the way for the followers of the ancients, they will learn to take the bit between their own teeth and steadfastly tread the trail to eternity, the bliss within the within-ness. Their torches are well fuelled and all that is required is someone to ignite the light which burns inside, blazing the route home to God, the Infinite, the Magnificent, the Greatest Creator of All. Then, when the work has reached the point when it manages itself, you, the earthly guides, will make a turning of your own choice either to move on to a new level, or give further support to the masses moving nearer to their Living God. You can choose how to live your own light in the firework display of all things. It is what God wants most, that you see the truth from your own perspective, with the God-spark within.

"And when this Day of Reckoning comes, you will see the Glow of God, and those who have done their introspective work will recognise this Glow and will not be afraid. You will no longer recognise the face of your mother, brother or child when you return to the halls of justice. All will have the same face, the face of Adam. The angels will sit on the footstool of the Eternal and Omniscient God and you will be your own judge. There will be the underscoring of your Book of Life and balance will be restored. I shall be there by your side, beseeching to the All Merciful God to forgive your sins, and you will resurrect into your third life. There is a place prepared for everyone following the End of Days. Mother Earth and the Heavenly Father will be tempered and flattened, and mankind will resurrect in accordance with his own deeds and choice of living.

"So, remember, my children, the whole world is only a footstool of the Lord God and God's eyes are everywhere."

Babaji smiled reassuringly and bid his disciples to take some evening food before leaving for the day. They had much food for thought before putting their heads down on their pillows that night.

Keeping Your Vehicle in Flow

When God created the universes and galaxies, He also made the gold, silver and red river-flows of life within each man, woman and child. These flows are the balancing of the sun, moon and mars. The sun is the heat, the fire; the moon is the cool, the water; and Mars is the work-horse which brings all living essence to the base and drives forward the beingness of mankind. Man will always want to progress while ever his red-flow is in motion. However, it is important to drive your inner vehicle with care as you manoeuvre the lessons and trials of earthly living.

The kriyas are the toolbox of balanced living. You can put your hand into the many layers of appropriate kriyas in order to keep your earthly vehicle in good shape. Here are eight basic kriyas for you to commence the servicing of your inner engine:

The Key of the Breath

It is important to understand about the key of the breath before commencing the kriyas. The key is situated at the soft place at the base of the throat, where the epiglottis is to be semi-closed in order to draw up the energy when doing the kriyas, much like a syringe draws up liquid. Before inhaling, ensure that the breath is emptied from the system, squeezing the navel area completely in. Keep your attention on the breath and when the inhalation is complete, turn your eyes up towards the centre of the brow at the third eye chakra. Really turn your eyes up as much as you are able and hold your attention at this spot. Here you will be in a position to 'see' yourself.

When sitting in the semi or full-lotus position, your arms should be fully extended and straight, resting the hands on your knees. There are a selection of mudras, hand positions, which can be used, such as the thumb to forefinger with the remaining digits held straight and closed together. Or you can place the thumb at the base of the little finger which is the earth element, or the ring-finger which is the air element. The best choice is simply to put the hands in a relaxed mode when first setting out with the kriyas. Gradually you can add to your toolbox of exercises.

1. Kapalabhati Kriya

Do this kriya to clear the nadis up and down. This cleanses the system of any obstruction before moving the energy up and down.

Sit in semi-lotus position with your spine erect and head in line with the back. Rest your hands gently on your knees with straight arms, and centre your attention on your breath. Breathe through your nose and pump the breath up and down, taking the breath into the chest cavity. Pull the stomach in and draw the shoulders up. On the exhale, let your shoulders drop down and push the stomach out. This breathing should be done with a fluid tempo for a minute or two, until you feel the highway is cleared. Enjoy the process of this cleansing exercise. It is a mantra of living to constantly work at all stages of your travel and it is to be relished.

2. Bhastrika Kriya

This breath clears the horizontal energies which can collect in the stomach area and works the opposite direction to that of the kapalabhati. It also begins the stoking up of the fire within, energising the kundalini at the mooladhara (base) chakra into action.

Take the breath in through the nose into the stomach area. Do not move the breath into the chest. Fill the stomach with the breath and then pump the breath out, using the muscles around the stomach with a positive movement inwards. Thus, the breath works in the mooladhara like a pair of bellows. This kriya can be done at a fast or slow pace, punching out the breath on the exhale. Again, do this exercise for as long as your body requires, until the energy feels vibrant throughout the whole system. You may feel dizzy, at which point relax and feel what the energy is doing in the different areas of your body. Keep your attention on your third eye and see your system thrive with the Breath of God within.

3. Right (Anuloma) and Left (Viloma) Nostril Breath

The right nostril takes in the heat or sun energy which is the gold flow, and the left nostril takes in the cool or moon energy which is the silver flow. You can adjust this kriya to whatever is required by your body, whether you need the heat or the cool.

Take the breath in through the right nostril up to the chest, without filling the stomach. You will need to hold your forefinger against the side of the left nostril to control the in-flowing breath into the right nostril until you are able to accomplish this kriya without doing so. Then let the breath out through the left nostril slowly, at the same energy level as the in-breath, moving the forefinger against the right nostril. Then inhale again by the left nostril and out through the right. This is one 'breath' and balances the energy systems within.

4. Soham Kriya

This kriya is to get the breathing process regularised as you proceed into full meditation. It will bring the energies into harmony around the chakras, awakening all elements of the constitution.

Draw the breath up with the mouth open, bringing it around the head, around the source of the Water of Life, and back down the front of the body on exhalation. See the energy move up and down, reverberating the spinning wheels of the chakras as you put the light matter where it will best do its work. The system is to be cranked up each time you do the kriyas and this kriya is an excellent tool with which to move down the gears of your vehicle.

5. The Bee Kriya

This kriya is a good one to do in order to get the flow of energy zinging around the bone structure of the whole body. For this you need to stand with the feet slightly apart and the knees slightly bent. Keep your spine straight and your head in alignment. Hold your arms out straight at 45º from your hips. Take a deep breath in (you can use the soham breath if you like) and when fully inhaled, turn your head to the right shoulder, rest the chin on the shoulder and exhale, making a buzzing sound between your teeth like a bee. Exhale completely and repeat the process down the left shoulder. This directs the energy down the arm, to the finger tips. It also resonates through the skull and down the spine, down the legs to the tips of the toes. See how the energy vibrates the full length of the body.

6. Circular Breath

This breath draws the energy up from the mooladhara chakra, up the spinal column, then pushes the energy flow up around the back of the head and over the forehead, flowing down the front of the body, down the rivers of life, back to the mooladhara. It is called the circular breath and is a method of moving energy throughout the system, bringing it past the top vertebrae from where you can extend into full meditation, when all consciousness of external noise and goings-on is lost and you are not aware of your breathing.

Sit in semi or full-lotus position with your arms extended straight out to your knees. You can use the mudra of thumb to base of ring-finger. Ensure that the breath is drawn up using the key at the base of the throat, and bring the energy up from the base chakra, up the spine. See the light energy spread up the spinal column along the nervous system, reaching all parts of the body. When the breath is fully inhaled, lock the key at the throat and push the energy up the back of the head and around to the top and front of the forehead. Turn your eyes up towards the third eye and hold the breath for as long as you are able. You can put the tip of your tongue at the soft part at the back of your pallet, which directs the energy up towards the higher realms, connecting you with God. Then push the energy down the front of the body (bring the tip of your tongue back down), expending all air out at the navel area.

7. Knocking and Churning

The churning kriya is when we churn the rivers of milk which flow from the head into the oceans of sorrow. It helps the process of separating the milk from the water by firstly making the milk into a curd, and eventually we make the curd into butter which no longer mixes with the waters of emotions. The knocking opens the doors which are closed, releasing the matter of our issues for introspection and healing.

Commence with the circular breathing, but draw the breath up, locking or knocking it at each chakra point from the mooladhara to the throat. You may draw the breath up approximately 30% before starting the knocking at the mooladhara, whichever way you are most comfortable with. Then lock the breath at the key and push the energy up at the back of the head, as with the circular breath. Hold the breath for a time before turning the head (left or right) in a full circle, taking care not to be too vigorous with the neck and top of the spine. Turn the head three times before bringing the breath back down, knocking at each of the chakras from the throat to the base. If you become short of breath, then take a continued breath in between the knocking breath to regain control and balance. It is best to do the churning only three or four times as it should be taken gently from the milk to the curd, to butter. The churning process is not to be hurried, but done with sure and steady movement.

8. The Silent Prayer

When your kriya practice has taken you to the level of consciousness when the body is beating with the Breath of God and your song is being sung, draw the breath up slowly, gently, holding the energy in rhythm with God's Breath as you climb to the top. Hold the breath and fall into the silence of God's Name, just being in the centre of His Loving Being. He will rejoice in your company and the heavens will ring out with angel trumpets blasting out the vibrations of all God's creation. His colours will reflect on your face, which will glow with all of God's qualities.

These are a sample of kriyas as given by Babaji, but it is always best to take instruction from an accomplished kriya master, who has been given the kriya initiation directly from Babaji. The energy of this yoga system is the highway to God and is just another of Babaji's gifts to those seeking enlightenment. The road to God-realisation is simple, but we are apt to make things more complex. Use the kriyas simply and enjoy the process of walking the Righteous Path, God's Path of the chosen beings.

The Divine Mother is Available to All

There are many visitors to Babaji's ashram from all parts of the globe. Some come with a specific thought in mind to search the way to God through the kriyas, and wish to be taught the techniques. Others just arrive in the midst of Babaji's aura wondering where they are meant to be going. They are the ones who are called by him to aid him with his mission, and are the messengers of his gospel. These messengers are all at different stages of their own path to enlightenment or, indeed, are the enlightened beings, come to show an example to the masses. Such enlightened beings are regular visitors to Babaji, who wish to follow the footsteps of previous masters and prophets, and are the selected ones to take mankind through his graveyard of errors and sin on Mother Earth. They will take the Seed of God in mankind into the realms of higher consciousness when the day of Armageddon arrives. The Seed of God will survive this day and the prophet, Jesus, will return shortly to see that punishment is meted out to those who declined God's Way, but took their own steps on earth towards the dense outer regions of the devil's domain.

There is a woman who lives in the very south of England. She is working the peace mission with the Dalai Lama, also a disciple of Babaji, and teaching the kriyas to those who seek the light. The teaching methods of this master are that of the Divine Mother, who shines through her smiling face. She glows with the Light of God and her eyes are the mirror in which to see your own God-consciousness. She is fully available to all who wish to learn the way to God. She teaches in simple terms and gives messages direct from her own Master, Babaji. She knows how he wills, and does his work with love and understanding. There are the stars in her eyes which are the geometry of life. They sparkle the hologram of Babaji's initiations into those who search and ask.

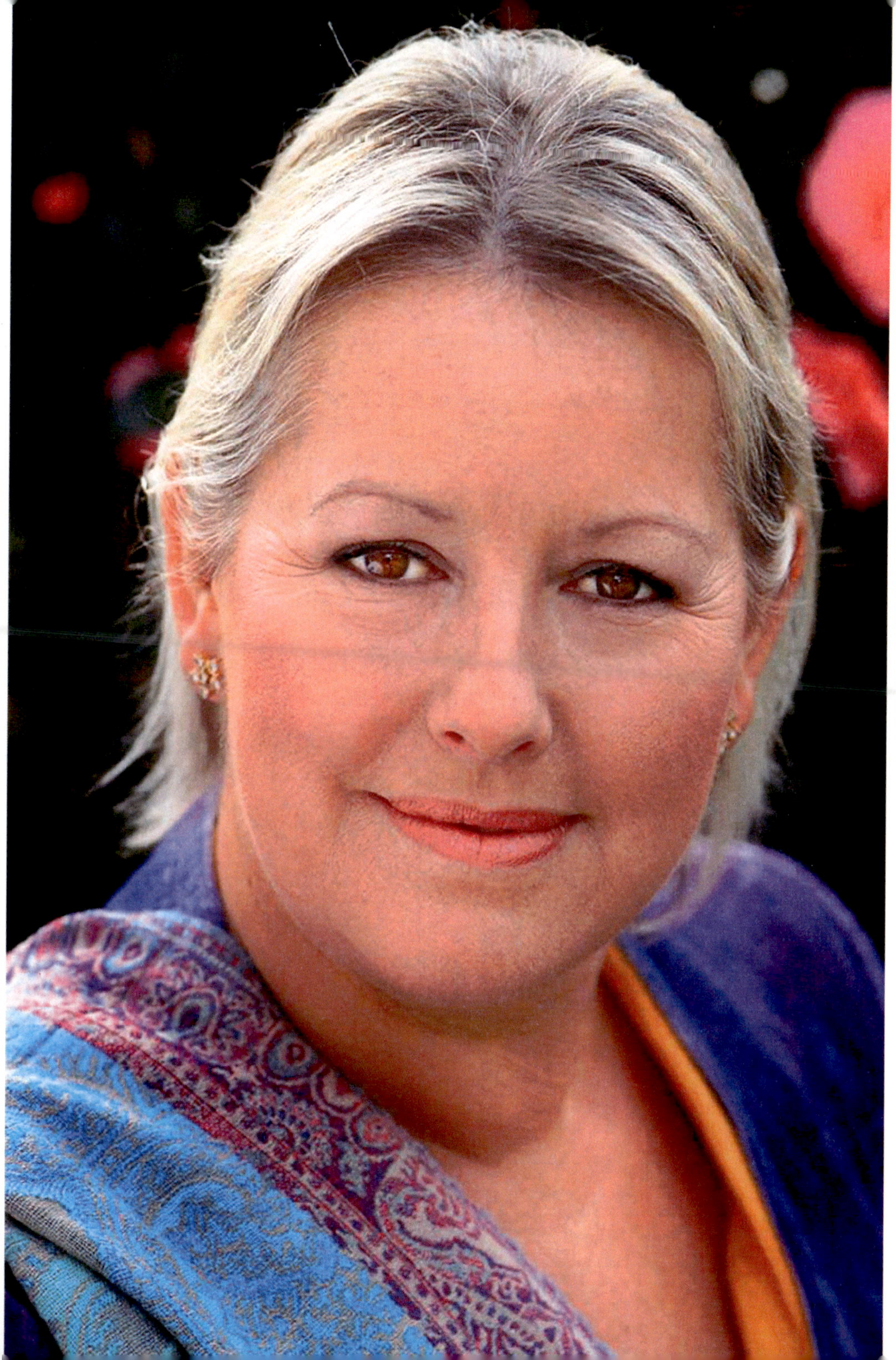

Many people are drawn to her side without knowing why, but stay for as long as possible. The vibration of this woman is so light and strong, the web enmeshes the most timid of souls to her midst. Babaji regards her as his shining light on the way to eternity, and has promised to lead the exodus into the fourth dimension through the network of such souls, here on earth to help the process of the resurrection. She will be by the side of Jesus when Babaji is no longer here, when his mission is completed. He says there will be no more prophets after him (Babaji is a messenger of God, a cry on the mountain for Jesus). This woman from England is a disciple of Jesus and will accomplish the work of his chosen ones assuredly.

The Mother of the Divine is in the logos of God's intention. Her essence is the head of the way of all things.

When a person comes on to earth with a mission such as this lady, then she is given the fast-track, advanced learner's method of accomplishing her starting point for this work. Her own lessons are no different from that of the next person, but the way she moves towards her goal is paramount to the enabling of those who choose to move with her. Therefore, she has been equipped with the soft but strong qualities of the Divine Mother and grounded it here on Mother Earth.

Her name is Paramahansa Aliyananda, named for the rejoicement of life that she is. Babaji gave her this name when she brought a group of potential chosen beings to see him, some eight years after she first found him in the mountains of Nainital. Her lessons were being learnt, but her master quality maintained her position by the side of Babaji, and this will be the quality which will see her by the side of her own followers. The kriyas are initiated through her to the listening ones who love and revere their master. Her kriya group which meets regularly in Penzance in Cornwall, as well as her own home in Penrose, receives the blessings of Babaji, and her words drop like gold from her mouth as she explains the godliness that is to be sought after. Her teachings come direct from Source with the watchful eye of Babaji at her shoulder, ensuring a direct hit with the gathering of people sitting in her midst.

Search this master out if the terrain in India is too much to see Babaji. Paramahansa Aliyananda is readily accessible and works in more central areas of the United Kingdom, as well as in her own County of Cornwall. She has a website which will come up on the internet if you type 'kriya yoga' into the search engine, or the address is www.kriyayoga.org.uk , e-mail aliyananda@hotmail.co.uk

Faith and Belief in The Living God

There are those who like to look at a beautifully sculptured statue of saintly beings when pouring out their troubles and woes. There are those who like to look at the sun and moon for Godly inspiration. They are both free to follow their own beliefs, of course, but the Essence of God is nearer than they are giving credence. He is the Almighty, Who is within them and without them. They are knocking at an external door when they bow down to their idols and outer stars of destiny. The way to go is within, not without, for the answers to their prayers.

God has ears and eyes everywhere. He knows every tiny secret which you hold in the smallest of rooms in your inner mansion. Let there be no doubting His presence when you are at your lowest ebb, when the earth is tilting so sharply that you feel you will fall off. He is there at your hour of need, ready to set you back on your feet in the direction back to Him. There is no doubting His Hand when He holds you in His Palm and says into your ear, "Thou that holdeth My Name as a shield and girdle will surely mete out the Love of God to those around. Thou hast no fear of living in My Realms of Righteousness, for the fear will dissipate into the ethers of the universe as the mists lift from your mountain tops. I shall deliver thee into the Kingdom of Heaven when the day of resurrection comes. Be thou of sure heart and mind when the time is nigh, for there will be those around you who shall look to thee for reassurance of My Existence. Be, therefore, a staff and rod, thyself, as a guide to those who only have the eyes for their own gods and limited destinies. Reassure them of the boundlessness of the Living God. I AM."

Babaji was putting together a potion of messages and healing for the day's visitors to his side. He wished that his people would recognise the path when it was placed before them, but not all were capable of daring to let go of their existing belief systems of man's own making throughout the ages. He could see the doubt rise into their faces when he related the truth. He was unrelenting with his message, however, and today he would pour each of them a tisane of elder, a floral essence to awaken the deepest of doubting souls. This was a remedy for the introspective traveller, who had reached a point of being stuck, but knew that the mire into which he had waded was only a temporary circumstance. The elder would dilute the bogs of sentiments and doubts, giving way to clearer understanding of life as it was intended by our Creator.

The potion was placed on the mantle above Babaji where the sun energy shone directly through the glass container, repotentising the stimuli of its contents. As he prepared the small drinking vessels for a ceremony of initiation for his disciples, he let the Name of God fall from his inner tongue, which also energised the healing properties of the liquid of elder essence. The potion was well potentised and all ready for the recipients, Babaji's messengers and gardeners.

He had called them to his side this day for a special ceremony of initiation, and he was to watch them carefully as they sat the test of faith and belief in the Living God. The love and devotion written in their faces was there for him to see as they took their chosen places for meditation. Some took cushions for comfort whilst sitting in the lotus position, and others merely maintained an upright spine whilst taking a seat on the outer edges of the meditation room. The inner sanctum was imbued with angelic presence as they wove their healing magic throughout the gathering. The golden energy of their light essence was inspiring.

"Let the light of the angels fill your body. Breathe them in as you begin the opening kriyas ready for deep meditation, children," began Babaji. "I want to deliver the Name of God to you, so that you can realise the Truth of His Eternity, so that you can increase your trust and belief in the One Omniscient Living God.

"You are all at different points of your individual journeys towards self-realisation and, ultimately, God-realisation. Allow this process to take its own time in its own natural rhythm in the Breath of God. You are alone in your quest to God-realisation, but there is support from all quarters. Call on your guides and personal 'made-easies' to ease the burden of life's trials and tribulations. They are there purely to light the way, to lead you through your own dark patches of spiritual growth, when the sun does not reach those certain places of shadow within. See the outstretched hands of the support system of your Creator, the All Merciful and Loving God. Feel the wings of those beings of light in and around you. Know the eyes of the Almighty God are watching your efforts when placing yourself at the mercy of His safety net. The Divine Father and Mother, too, have a vested interest in your progress along the winding path of inner struggle. Be transparent and trust that the end result will be uncluttered with the heavy burden of man's efforts at earthly existence. Life is simple and need not be encumbered with the baggage of travelling in synthetic mode. Keep things in divine order in your life and take each step with ease."

Babaji gave each person a small cup of elder, which they drank whilst in communication with their God. They felt the liquid move to the third eye, expanding the introspective process as they began the kriya breathing. He watched as they did this, as the light of the angels began to build up in the room. He waited for a full hour before leading the group into a space where they had not dared to venture before. The boundaries were being stretched and this was always uncomfortable. The feeling of not

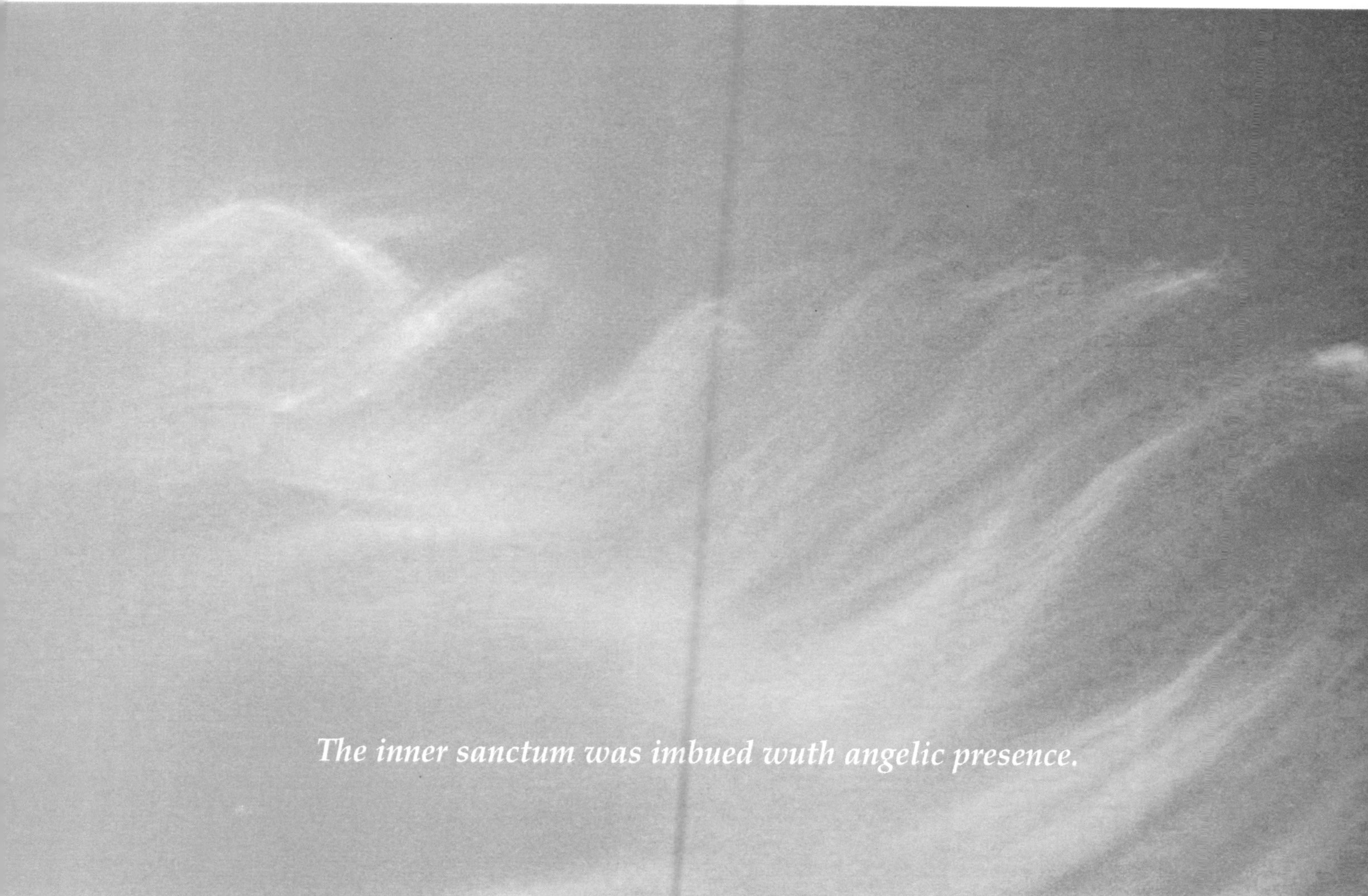

The inner sanctum was imbued wuth angelic presence.

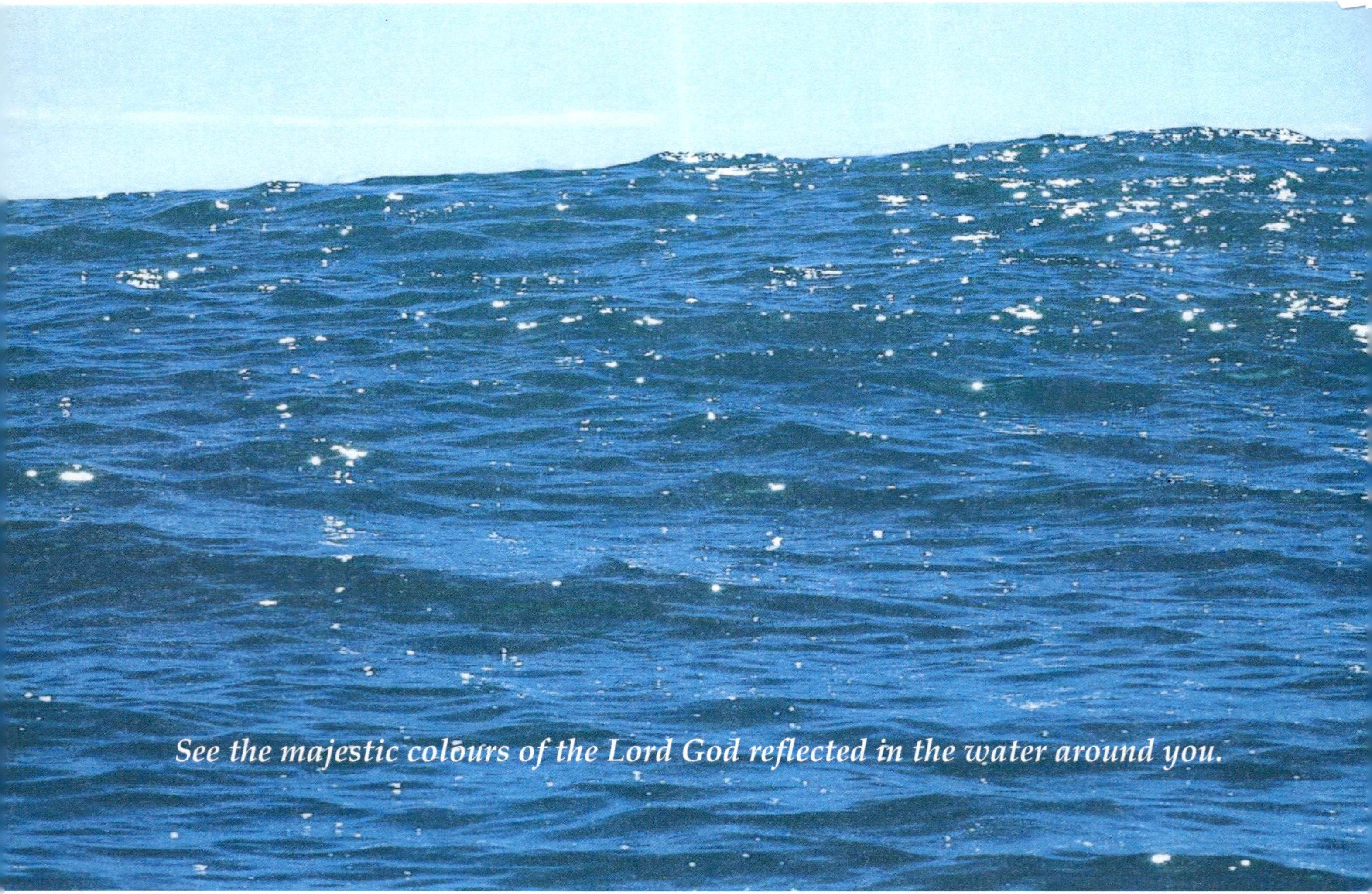

See the majestic colours of the Lord God reflected in the water around you.

being safe was a part of the human's psyche, and the support system was there to take away this fear. The fears of the group, of course, were varied, but their Master knew each and every issue of his disciples.

"The ocean waters are a little rough now, but look ahead at the horizon. The sun is radiating its light on the smooth tides of change. Allow the sails of your vessel to take the breeze, which will bring you to your own horizon where you can observe all islands visited. Leave behind the uncertainties of the mindset given to you through worldly experiences. Now see the majestic colours of the Lord God reflected in the water around you. Your vessel is strong and leaks no issues in. You can appreciate the power of the water's swell, moving you towards the diamond star on the rim of the horizon. Nothing is insurmountable, and your heart is filled with the knowingness of success. On the horizon there is a galleon waiting for you. Its sails are billowing in the wind you will be given the courage to step from your small sailing boat, first with one foot and, more importantly, then with the second foot. Dare to leave the cocoon of life as you know it, into the plains of spiritual living where there are no obstacles of fear or unharmonious energies around you. You are in complete harmony with the Breath of God and the galleon is God's Vessel, come to collect you from your false haven. The path is clear to walk, and the footfall of your dreamy self is but a fraction of a millimetre away from being established in the fullest flow of God's Own Living Name. Once you have set yourself upon the decks of God's galleon, then feel the elixir of the sun's energies filling your cup. This cup will never be empty, but constantly overflowing with the Love of God, teaming down your own river waters of life, cleansing and purifying.

"Have faith and belief in the Love of the Living God. Have faith in the abundance of the Dharma, the Path of Righteousness. Believe in the surety of God's Way. He will not allow you to fall. You have His assurance and it is the Way of All Things. Move yourself out of the insecurities of mankind's worldly desires and quick-fixes, into the eternal realms of immortality."

The Master blessed each one with an opportunity to reach this state of being, and left the meditation room to continue his work with his patients who were patiently waiting outside for his ministering. How easily he moved from one need of his people to another. His energy was limitless on the prana of God's Breath.

A Letter to a Friend

Nainital
October 2006

Dear Angela,

May this letter bring you birthday wishes and blessings from Babaji, here in Nainital. He blew his message of God's Living to you, so that you can shine the Glow of God on to those who come to you for the tender loving care of the Divine Mother. You are blessed with the grandness of heart which ministers to those in need. Show them the path, the Way of God. Show them the ease of the way. Let thy light illuminate the simplicity of the art of living, even in the dark streets of man's construction.

Be of good cheer that Mother Earth is managing her own breathing process. God is her Creator, too, and He shall not fail her. He sends his messengers and gardeners, the chosen beings, to help with the tending of her fields, meadows and rivers of life, which flow into the oceans of God's Almighty Waters. The seas are the heavens and we are sailing the tides. The tides are the vehicle of His Path, and man cannot stop this ultimate power. He is the Greatest Creator of All and man is on the brink of the highest wave ever. He will be taken to the sea-shore with the certainty of All That Is, there to venture on the inroads of his own wisdom within. God is within him, too, and he is a star of unique quality. Only with God's Grace can he make his every step along the highway to God-realisation.

So, my sister, my love wings its way to you in England from India. Feel the blessings of Babaji whoosh out as you open the seal of this letter. The course of time is in divine order and you are growing more beautiful as the days pass by. He says to tell you that if you so wish, a journey to your mountain in the Himalayas, Mount Annapurna, can be arranged. He will take you on a journey of a lifetime into the very heart of its standing. Here you will feel God's Breath even in the density of the hard rock of the

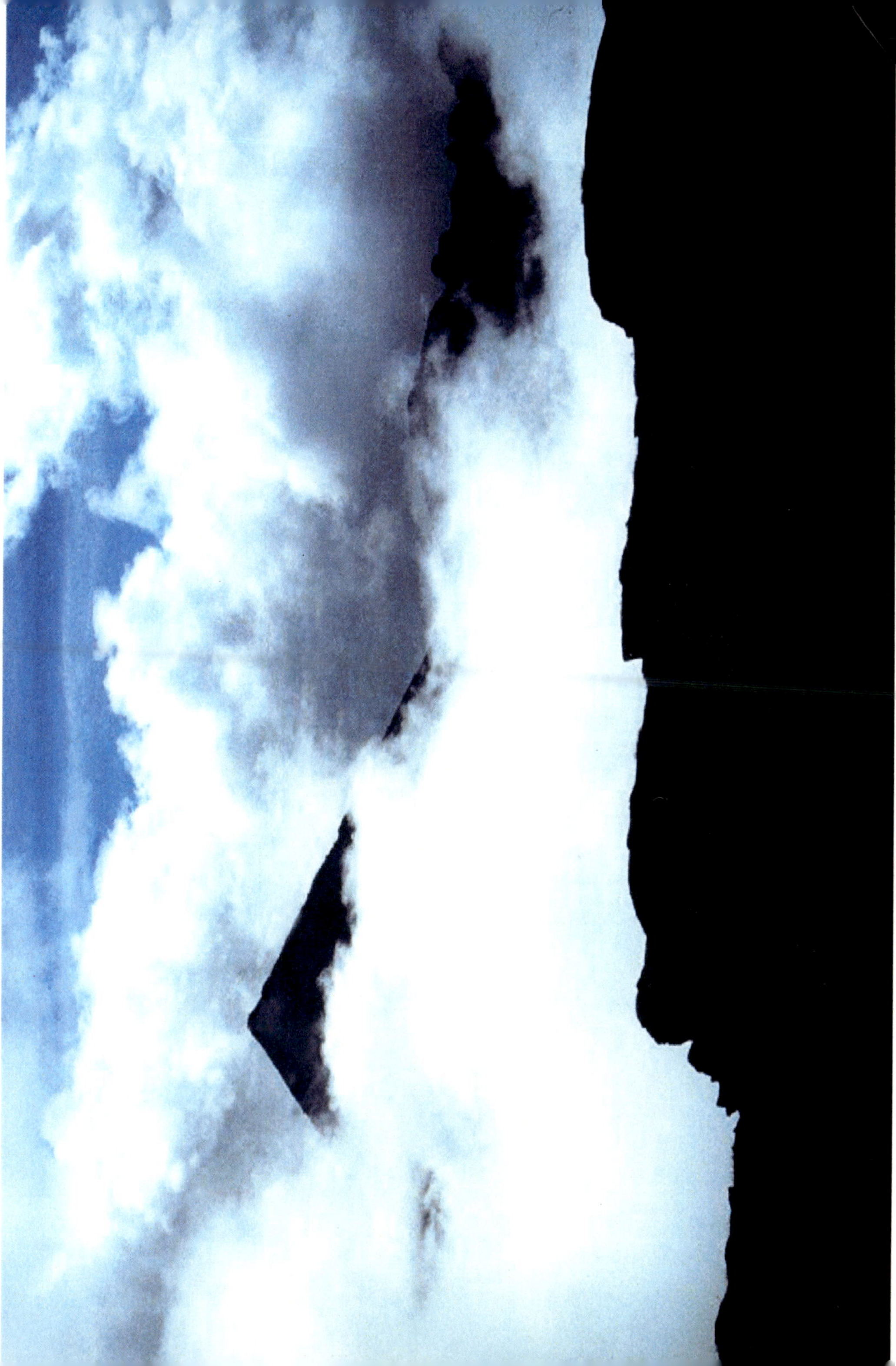

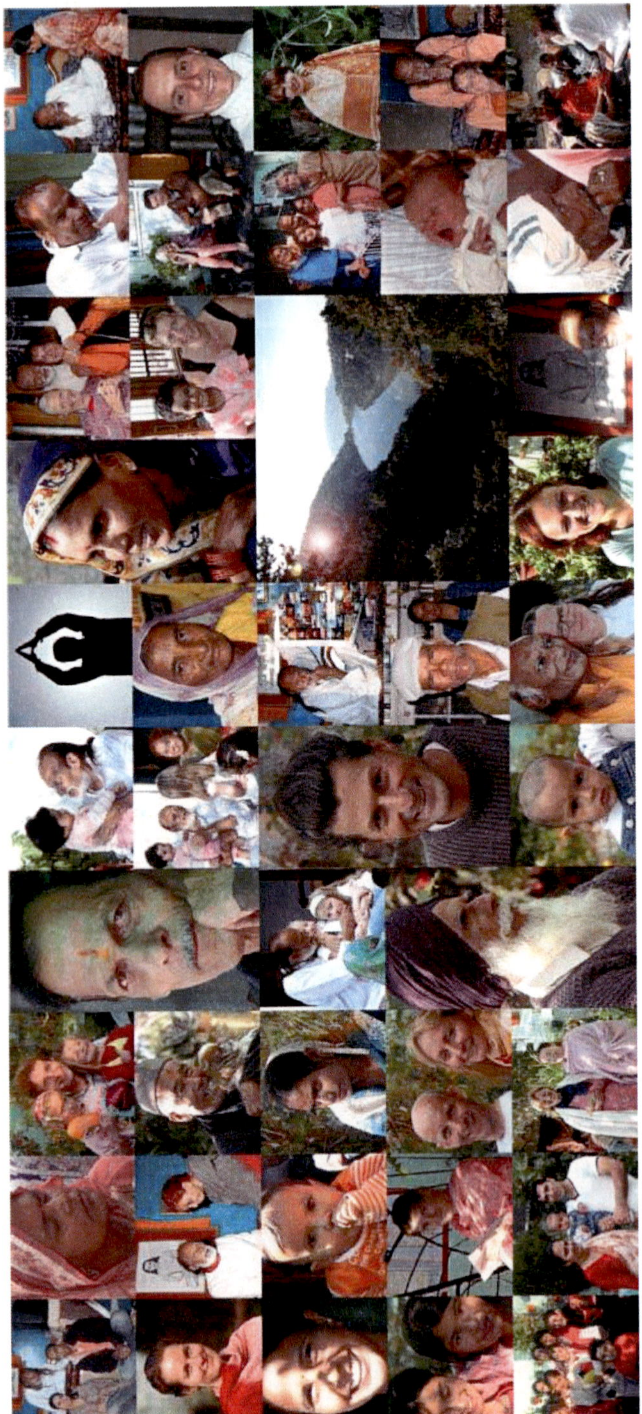